Nutrition
A Beginner's Guide

ONEWORLD BEGINNER'S GUIDES combine an original, inventive, and engaging approach with expert analysis on subjects ranging from art and history to religion and politics, and everything in-between. Innovative and affordable, books in the series are perfect for anyone curious about the way the world works and the big ideas of our time.

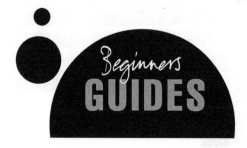

Nutrition
A Beginner's Guide

Dr Sarah Brewer

ONEWORLD

A Oneworld Book

Published by Oneworld Publications 2013

Copyright © Sarah Brewer 2013

The moral right of Sarah Brewer to be identified as the Author
of this work has been asserted by her in accordance with
the Copyright, Designs and Patents Act 1988

ISBN 978-1-85168-924-8
ISBN (ebook) 978-1-78074-081-2

Typeset by Cenveo, India
Printed and bound in Great Britain by
TJ International Ltd, Cornwall.

Oneworld Publications
10 Bloomsbury Street
London WC1B 3SR
UK

This book is dedicated to my wonderful family, who provide love and support during all those long hours of research and writing!

Contents

Tables and diagrams

[*] © Crown copyright. Department of Health in association with the Welsh Assembly Government, the Scottish Government and the Food Standards Agency in Northern Ireland.
[†] © U.S. Department of Agriculture. MyPyramid.gov website. Washington, DC.

Introduction: do you live to eat or eat to live?

When it comes to food, do you follow Hippocrates' famous axiom: 'You are what you eat' and select the most healthy, nutritious diet possible? Or do you follow the advice of Mark Twain: 'Eat what you like and let the food fight it out inside'?

Each of us has a complex relationship with food that goes beyond obtaining the nutrition required to fuel growth, body maintenance, physical activity and good health. Some live only to eat – planning meals and snacks in advance, experimenting with new tastes and craving old favourites. These people are likely to obtain more nutrition than they need and struggle with weight-related health issues. But some eat only to live, juggling their body image and hunger to obtain just enough nutrition to sustain life. Interestingly, the way you obtain nutrition can have a huge impact on your health, and even your life expectancy. For example, prolonged calorie restriction has been shown to extend average lifespan by 50 to 100 per cent in all species studied, including yeast, worms, spiders, flies, fish, mice, rats, dogs and monkeys. In all likelihood, a restricted diet can extend human life, too. In fact, according to a recent review from the Pennington Biomedical Research Center, cutting back on food intake (while maintaining proper nutrition to guard against vitamin and mineral deficiencies) is the only intervention known to slow consistently the rate at which we age and to increase the human lifespan. So what's the catch? Well, cutting back on food intake isn't as easy as it sounds – as any calorie-controlled dieter will tell you. And you need to restrict calories to around two-thirds of your normal daily needs in order to prolong your life by twenty to forty years. Yet while a so-called starvation diet may be associated with a longer lifespan, more often than not it is accompanied by protein and micronutrient deficiencies that attract their own health problems.

The ideal is to strive for balance, so that you live to eat, as well as eat to live.

This book necessarily concentrates on the 'eat to live' side of the equation, exploring why you need macronutrients (carbohydrate, protein, fat, fibre) and micronutrients (vitamins, minerals, trace elements, phytochemicals) in your diet. It explains how food is digested and metabolized to obtain energy, and how it provides the building blocks for your body's growth and repair. It looks at how much energy you need to fuel your basal metabolic rate – the amount of energy you burn at rest to maintain normal body functions – and physical activity levels, and even touches on weight maintenance and weight-loss diets. It offers a variety of detailed nutritional guidelines and shows you how optimal health can be achieved through the right nutritional balance.

The link between diet and health was suspected thousands of years ago. Hippocrates, a Greek physician born around 460 BC, was famous for quotes such as: 'Let food be your medicine, and medicine be your food.' It was only in 1747, however, that James Lind conducted the first controlled experiment to show that a disease – scurvy – resulted from a dietary deficiency. Although Lind's findings on scurvy were accepted at the time, it took forty years before the Admiralty ordered ships to receive a supply of lemon or lime juice, which helped eradicate scurvy from the Royal Navy. This is perhaps the first illustration of how slowly nutritional guidelines tend to change to keep up with published science.

FINDING A CURE FOR SCURVY

On voyages of exploration during the sixteenth and seventeenth centuries, as many as 90 per cent of sailors died from scurvy. In 1747, naval surgeon James Lind discovered that oranges and lemons could cure scurvy in a controlled trial aboard his ship, HMS *Salisbury*.

In his publication *A Treatise of the Scurvy* (1753), he reported: 'I took 12 patients in the scurvy . . . putrid gums, the spots and lassitude, with weakness of their knees. They . . . had one diet common to all . . . Two were ordered each a quart of cider a day. Two others took . . . elixir vitriol three times a day, using a gargle strongly acidulated with it for their mouths. Two others took two spoonfuls of vinegar three times a day, upon an empty stomach, having their gruels and other food well acidulated with it, as also the gargle for their mouth. Two of the worst patients . . . were put under a course of sea-water. Of this, they drank half a pint every day . . . Two others had each two oranges and one lemon given them every day. These they ate with greediness, upon an empty stomach. They continued but six days under this course, having consumed the quantity that could be spared. The two remaining patients took . . . an electuary recommended by an hospital-surgeon, made of garlic, mustard-seed, rad. Raphan, balsam of Peru and gum myrrh; using for common drink, barley-water well acidulated with tamarinds . . . The consequence was, that the most sudden and visible good effects were perceived from the use of the oranges and lemons; one of those who had taken them, being at the end of six days fit for duty. The other was the best recovered of any in his condition; and being now deemed pretty well, was appointed nurse to the rest of the sick.'

More recently, the link between diet and health – or lack of it – has become better understood, partly as a result of population-based observational studies. However, observational studies can only show an association – they do not provide definite proof. Correlations have been observed between the annual stork population in the Netherlands and the human birth rate, for example, but this does not prove that babies are delivered by storks. Interesting observations must therefore be followed up with trials specifically designed to test a particular hypothesis. These trials should, ideally, be:

- randomized (participants are randomly allocated to one or other groups)
- placebo-controlled (one group receives the active test treatment, while another group receives an inactive dummy treatment).
- double-blind (neither investigators nor participants know who is getting the true treatment, and who receives the dummy treatment)

Such double-blind, randomized, placebo-controlled trials are considered the gold standard for all academic research, including nutritional studies. The outcomes of those taking the active treatment are then compared with those taking a placebo and compared statistically. If the probability of the observed result occurring by chance alone is less than 5 per cent, the finding is considered statistically significant. This means that, in any one trial, there is still a chance, however small, that the 'statistically significant' result was due to chance alone. As a result, the concept of a meta-analysis has been developed, in which the findings from many similar studies are pooled together and the combined results compared statistically. This helps to balance out those findings, both positive and negative, that are due to chance and to give a more accurate assessment.

Another approach is to use a systematic review, in which a literature search identifies all high-quality research trials relating to a particular question to provide an exhaustive overview of the evidence base. These systematic reviews may also use statistical techniques such as meta-analysis to combine the results of the eligible studies. Where possible, the results of these larger analyses are included in this book to show the strength of evidence to support particular nutritional pearls of wisdom.

Changing your diet can have a massive impact on your health. To ensure that these changes and impacts are beneficial rather than detrimental, an abundance of scientific evidence is needed before nutrition scientists and governments are confident that new recommendations or guidelines are needed. This slow pace can seem frustrating at times. For example, in the 1990s, the recommendation for pregnant women to take folic acid supplements helped to cut the number of babies born with neural tube defects, such as spina bifida, by around 70 per cent. But the debate about whether or not to fortify flour with folic acid (to protect the babies of women who do not take supplements) is still continuing over twenty years later, as this would also increase intakes of folic acid for another sector of the population – the elderly – for whom folic acid supplementation could mask the red blood cell changes needed to help detect vitamin B12 deficiency. If left undiagnosed, a severe lack of B12 could lead to pernicious anaemia and a form of irreversible nerve damage known as subacute combined degeneration of the spinal cord.

This neatly illustrates why an exact understanding of nutrition is so important in order to do good while avoiding harm.

The ins and outs of digestion

The food you eat provides energy, building blocks and vital nutrients – preferably locked up in delicious morsels. Before you can access these benefits, the food must be broken down into its simplest components and absorbed across your intestinal wall into your circulation.

Good nutrition depends on the proper functioning of your gastrointestinal tract, or gut, which forms a coiled tube around 9 metres in length. Complex food molecules are inserted at one end and worn down into simpler, soluble components through a combination of mechanical and chemical disruption – a process known as digestion. Valuable nutrients are then absorbed, while unwanted waste products are disposed of, usually in neat packages, at the other end.

The mouth

Digestion starts in your mouth. Food is mechanically disrupted by the biting, chewing and tearing action of your teeth. At the same time, saliva moistens food with powerful enzymes (molecules that trigger chemical reactions and speed them up); salivary amylase starts to dissolve the chemical bonds in starch, while salivary lipase starts digesting fats. A few other enzymes are also present, such as lysozyme and peroxidase to help kill bacteria – although as anyone who's ever suffered from food poisoning will know, these aren't always effective. Your tongue then rolls the moistened food into a ball and pushes it to the back of the mouth. This triggers the swallowing reflex (deglutition) and the bolus of food is pushed down into your stomach by a wave of muscular contraction.

FROM BLAND TO SWEET

You produce between 750 ml and 1,500 ml saliva per day. If you hold a starchy food such as bread in your mouth for any length of time, it will start to taste sweet as salivary amylase attacks starch molecules to release the sugar, maltose.

The stomach

Your stomach is a hollow, J-shaped muscular sac in the upper left-hand side of your abdomen, just beneath the diaphragm. Its inner surface is deeply folded, so it can 'shrink' when empty and expand after a large meal to hold as much as 2 litres of fluid at any one time. In fact, your stomach is the most elastic part of your body as it can stretch up to 50 times its empty size. The muscular walls of your stomach act like a concrete mixer, churning food and mixing it with gastric juices, of which you secrete around 3 litres per day.

THE 'JUICIER' THE BETTER

Stomach juices contain hydrochloric acid and two main enzymes: pepsin, which digests proteins into smaller protein chains called peptides, and gastric lipase, which breaks down dietary fats. Around 20 per cent of the lipase in your stomach comes from your saliva, which builds up in your stomach as you swallow between meals. To prevent the stomach from digesting itself, cells in the wall secrete mucin and bicarbonate, which line the stomach with a thick, alkaline, barrier gel. Stomach-lining cells are also shed and replaced every three to six days.

Depending on a meal's composition, it takes from two to six hours for your stomach to convert food into a semi-digested, creamy slurry known as chyme. Wave-like contractions then start to push the stomach contents down towards the stomach's exit, which is guarded by a powerful ring of muscle, the pyloric sphincter. This relaxes momentarily to allow small amounts of chyme to squirt into the first part of your small intestines, the duodenum. As more and more chyme passes through the pylorus and out of your stomach, your stomach gradually shrinks in size.

Small intestines

Your small intestines consist of three consecutive parts: the duodenum, jejunum and ileum. These form a highly coiled tube which, if fully stretched out, would measure 6 metres or more in length. High muscular tone in their walls constricts them down to half this length, however, so that they fit neatly into your abdominal cavity.

Your duodenum is a curved, C-shaped tube that encircles the head of the pancreas. It is around 25 cm long and secretes alkaline juices that neutralize the acidic chyme received from the stomach. This change in acid level is important both to avoid irritating the lining of your small intestines, and to help the next set of digestive enzymes work more efficiently. The duodenum also acts as the meeting place where chyme is introduced to the powerful actions of pancreatic juice and liver bile.

PANCREATIC JUICES

Secretions from the pancreas gland contain powerful enzymes that break down the chemical bonds in protein (trypsin, chymotrypsin, elastase), carbohydrates (amylase), fats (lipase, phospholipase) and nucleic acids (nucleases). Unlike herbivores, humans lack the enzymes needed to break down cellulose in plant walls and, instead, rely on the bacteria in the large bowel to help do this for us. Bile made in the liver is stored in the gall bladder. When food leaves the stomach, hormone signals cause the gall bladder to contract. Bile is then squirted down into the duodenum where it acts like a detergent, disrupting dietary fats to form small globules, which hastens their digestion by providing a greater surface area on which your digestive enzymes can get to work.

By the time food leaves your duodenum, complex molecules are almost fully digested and ready for absorption in the next part of the small intestines, your jejunum: long protein chains have been cleaved to release simpler units called peptides and amino acids; carbohydrates have disintegrated into sugars known as saccharides; triglyceride fats have split to release their glycerol backbone and fatty-acid tails.

The next part of your small intestines is where absorption occurs (although some substances such as alcohol and many drugs can be absorbed across the lining of the stomach or even the mouth). The small intestine below the duodenum consists of the jejunum, followed by the ileum. There is no distinct border between these two areas, and this division is somewhat arbitrary, with the jejunum consisting of around 40 per cent of the remaining small intestine, and the ileum 60 per cent. In general, the ileum is paler in colour than the jejunum, as its walls contain immune areas (Peyer's patches) that help to protect against food-borne infections.

ENZYMES AND SUBSTRATES

An enzyme is a special protein that speeds up a chemical reaction, which, without the enzyme, either would not occur at all, or would occur too slowly to be of any use. The substance on which the enzyme acts is known as its 'substrate'.

The jejunum and ileum secrete a fluid known as *succus entericus*. These juices contain enzymes that complete the digestive process in which your food is broken down into simpler chemicals ready for absorption into your body. Put succinctly:

- sucrase cleaves sucrose (table sugar, a disaccharide) to release glucose and fructose
- lactase breaks down lactose (milk sugar) to release glucose and galactose
- peptidases act on any remaining peptides to release their constitutive amino acids
- lipase continues the digestion of triglycerides into free fatty acids and glycerol.

So far in its journey through your intestines, food has been mechanically chewed and churned, then attacked with chemicals and enzymes to form a porridge-like slurry. This slurry is teeming with valuable sources of energy (especially sugars and fatty acids), protein building blocks (amino acids) and micronutrients ready for absorption.

The inner lining of the jejunum and ileum is ideally suited for this task as it is covered in finger-like projections (villi), which are between 0.5 mm and 2 mm in length.

Compared with a flat surface, these villi increase the surface area over which absorption can occur by a factor of 30. The villi within the lining of the jejunum are longer than those within the ileum, as this is where most nutrients are absorbed.

Water-soluble nutrients, such as amino acids and sugars, are taken up by tiny blood capillaries within the villi and sent, via the hepatic portal vein, straight to the liver for processing: amino acids are reassembled to form proteins such as clotting factors, while excess glucose is converted into fats or glycogen for storage.

In contrast, fatty substances such as fatty acids and cholesterol have to be repackaged to make them soluble before they can enter the bloodstream. This repackaging occurs in the intestinal lining cells on the surface of the villi. Known as enterocytes, these cells wrap fatty acids and cholesterol with special proteins to form soluble particles (chylomicrons) that are released into small lymph vessels (lacteals) within the villi itself. Then, rather than going to the liver, they travel via the lymphatic system to be released into the subclavian vein under the collarbone. As these chylomicrons travel around the body, some are broken down by enzymes (lipase) found in the circulation to release fatty acids that can be used as a fuel by body cells (especially in your heart and skeletal muscle), or stored in fat cells (adipocytes). Those that reach the liver are further processed and repackaged – for example, excess dietary saturated fats are converted into cholesterol.

THE COMPLEXITY OF VITAMIN B12 UPTAKE

Before it can be absorbed in the last part of the ileum, vitamin B12 must be bound to a substance called gastric intrinsic factor, which is secreted by specialized cells in the stomach lining. As you get older, you tend to produce less intrinsic factor, so that less vitamin B12 is absorbed. This can lead to a B12 deficiency that is associated with a pernicious anaemia and a number of neurological symptoms, such as muscle weakness. Severe lack of B12 can also lead to irreversible damage to the spinal cord, and dementia.

Between them, the jejunum and ileum process 9 to 10 litres of fluid per day; 2 to 3 litres from your diet, and 7 to 8 litres of digestive juices. Absorption is so efficient, however, that only 1 to 2 litres of fluid are left to pass through the ileocaecal valve that marks the end of the small intestines and the start of the large bowel.

Large intestines

The large bowel acts as a waste-packaging unit for the body. Around 1 metre long, it mainly consists of the colon and rectum. At the start is a blind-ending pouch, into which the ileum protrudes to act like a one-way valve. An increase in pressure in the small intestine allows the valve to open, while increases in pressure in the large bowel squeezes it closed. The appendix, which branches off from the first part of the large bowel (caecum), was long considered an evolutionary remnant (vestigial organ), but new research suggests it does play a useful yet non-essential role. It acts as a reservoir of 'friendly' gut bacteria that can readily repopulate the bowel after a bout of food poisoning, or after a course of antibiotics (which can kill beneficial bacteria as well as those associated with infection).

The colon absorbs fluid, salts and minerals from bowel contents. It also contains a trillion digestive bacteria – more than the number of human cells in your body. These bacteria ferment dietary fibre and synthesize nutrients such as vitamin K, biotin and folic acid, which you can absorb and use. Of around 2 litres of bowel contents received into the colon each day, on average only 10 per cent is voided as semi-solid waste.

Intestinal contractions

Once you swallow a mouthful of food, you have no further voluntary control on how it progresses through your intestines.

Bowel contents are propelled forward by waves of muscular contractions known as peristalsis and, while involuntary (in that they occur without you thinking about them), they are beautifully coordinated by the action of special receptors and hormone signals that detect when food is present. These peristaltic waves pass through your duodenum and jejunum at a frequency of around twelve contractions per minute – about as often as you breathe in and out at rest. In the ileum, the wave slows to around nine times per minute as fluid is absorbed and the volume of intestinal contents decreases. Peristalsis within the colon occurs at between two and six contractions per minute.

Ring-like segmentation contractions also occur in the gut at regular intervals, which move intestinal contents (chyme) to and fro so that as many nutrients as possible come into contact with the bowel wall for absorption.

A third type of contraction only occurs in the colon – the so-called mass action contraction. This constriction causes a large area of the colon to push the relatively dry waste material that remains after absorption of nutrients and fluid into the rectum. Rectal filling and distension then trigger the desire to open your bowels (defaecation reflex).

Normally, your absorptive processes are so efficient that most of the 'waste' reaching your colon consists of undigested dietary fibre. This is fermented by bowel bacteria to produce some useful nutrients, such as short-chain fatty acids (which you can absorb and use as a fuel). In fact, over half the weight of your stools consists of these bacteria!

CHOLECYSTOKININ (CCK)

As food distends the stomach, a hormone called cholecystokinin (CCK) is secreted into the duodenum. This causes the colon to contract and often brings on a strong desire to open the bowels (gastrocolic reflex). This is why babies often fill their nappies as they feed. CCK also plays a role in appetite control, as discussed later.

The liver

Your liver deserves a special mention as, like a major warehouse, it plays a vital role in processing and distributing the nutrients you absorb from your food. The liver is located in the upper part of your abdomen, just below the diaphragm, with the main bulk on the right-hand side.

The liver is unique in that it receives two separate blood supplies. Water-soluble nutrients absorbed from your intestines into your circulation pass directly to the liver within the hepatic portal vein. Dietary fats take a more convoluted route. First, they are made soluble within the lining cells of your small intestine, then absorbed via the lymphatic system as described earlier. Those that are not immediately taken up by muscle or fat cells then reach the liver within the hepatic artery. Once in the liver, blood from the hepatic portal vein and hepatic artery mingle within relatively large spaces (sinusoids) from which the liver cells extract the oxygen and nutrients.

The highly specialized cells where the main work of the liver is carried out are called hepatocytes. As well as secreting bile (which aids the digestion of fat in the duodenum), liver cells have many other important nutritional roles, such as:

- making proteins from amino acids
- converting ammonia, a waste product of amino-acid metabolism, into urea
- making glucose from glycerol, lactic acid and certain amino acids (e.g. alanine)
- storing excess glucose as glycogen – a starchy emergency fuel
- processing fatty acids to make triglycerides and cholesterol
- storing fat-soluble vitamins (A, D, E and K plus vitamin B12) and some minerals (e.g. iron and copper)
- filtering out foreign proteins carried from the intestines to reduce their impact on the immune system and allergies

- removing and detoxifying dietary poisons (e.g. alcohol)
- generating heat to warm passing blood and help regulate your metabolic rate.

So far, we have considered the perfect scenario in which foods are digested and absorbed when the gut is in perfect working order. However, there are times when food processing doesn't go so smoothly. If bowel contents pass through the intestinal tract too rapidly (for example, due to food poisoning, or excessive stress), nutrient and water absorption is incomplete resulting in diarrhoea. If this is prolonged, it can lead to dehydration, lack of energy and salt imbalances that can be life-threatening.Worldwide, diarrhoeal disease is the second leading cause of death in children under the age of five (after pneumonia). At the other end of the scale (for example, due to lack of dietary fibre, or the effects of morphine-related painkillers), bowel contents may pass through too slowly, so that excessive water is absorbed and wastes become dry and difficult to pass. Constipation can have a profound effect on your quality of life, and is a contributory cause of volvulus in which the bowel twists round on itself, provoking a surgical emergency.

Malabsorption can also develop, in which certain nutrients are not absorbed properly. Examples include lactose intolerance, due to insufficient production of the enzyme lactase, needed to digest milk sugar (lactose); coeliac disease, in which a type of gluten protein found in wheat causes an immune reaction that damages the lower jejunum; and an inability to digest and absorb dietary fats (which can have a number of causes such as lack of bile or pancreatic enzymes, to inflammatory bowel disease). Similarly, an inability to absorb vitamin B12 in the ileum can be due to lack of intrinsic factor (produced in the stomach to assist B12 absorption), or disease of the ileum itself.

Assuming digestion and absorption go as planned, however, the body receives a plentiful supply of both macronutrients (protein, carbohydrates, fat) and micronutrients (vitamins, minerals and trace elements) to meet its needs. The next chapter looks at macronutrients and what we do with them.

2

Getting down to basics: macronutrients

Just as you have to fill your car with petrol, diesel or, increasingly, plug it into an electricity supply, you need food to fuel your energy requirements. Energy is the dynamic force that underpins all your biological processes from growth, metabolism and reproduction to physical and mental exertion. Even digestion and absorption themselves require energy for chewing, secreting digestive enzymes, propelling food through the gut and transporting nutrients around the body. The extra workload of the liver also generates heat, and it is estimated that at least 10 per cent of the total energy yield of a meal is used up during its processing.

The energy in food is provided by three broad categories of chemicals – proteins, carbohydrates and fats. They have other roles too, of course. Proteins also act as building blocks for making enzymes and body tissues, while fats are an important component of cell membranes and are used to make hormones as well as regulating inflammation in the body. Even carbohydrates, which used to be thought of in terms of pure energy, are now known to be involved in the biological signalling that tells cells what to do.

Dietary proteins

Proteins form the basic structural units of your body. But as we have seen, the human body cannot absorb them in their complete form. First they must be digested down into their basic building blocks before absorption can take place. These building blocks are then used by your cells to make all the different human proteins in your body including antibodies, blood-clotting factors, cell receptors, transport proteins, lean muscle tissue and the collagen and elastin in your skin, cartilage and ligaments.

The building blocks within dietary proteins are called amino acids. These are linked together to form different chain lengths: chains containing between two and ten amino acids are known as peptides; those containing ten to 100 amino acids are called polypeptides; chains of over 100 amino acids, which fold into complex three-dimensional shapes, are known as proteins.

Protein digestion starts in your stomach when the enzyme pepsin cleaves the links in proteins and polypeptides to produce short peptide chains. Once in your small intestine, these are further attacked by enzymes released from the intestinal wall and pancreas. Some chains of double and triple amino acids (dipeptides and tripeptides) are absorbed into your gut lining cells (enterocytes), where they are broken apart to release single amino acids into the bloodstream.

Twenty-one amino acids are important for human health. Twelve of these can be synthesized from other building blocks within your own cells, but the remaining nine must come from your diet and are known as the nutritionally essential amino acids. These are: histidine, isoleucine, leucine, lysine, methionine, phenylalanine, threonine, tryptophan and valine.

On average, you need to obtain around 1 gram of dietary protein per day for each kilogram of your body weight. Someone weighing 70 kg, therefore, needs to obtain roughly 70 g of protein per day from their diet. This represents about 15 per cent of daily energy intake.

Dietary proteins originating from animals (meat, fish, eggs and dairy products) contain significant quantities of all the essential amino acids. Vegetable sources of protein (rice, beans, nuts, seeds) each contain some, but not all, of the essential amino acids.

Within a vegetarian diet, eating a variety of plant products is important to ensure a balanced intake of essential amino acids.

When your diet is rich in protein, excess amino acids cannot be stored in their original form. Instead, excess protein that is not needed for immediate growth or repair of body tissues is used directly as a fuel for energy, converted into glucose or, if energy is plentiful, converted into energy stores for later use.

ENERGY STORES

Starchy glycogen, which is stored in your liver and muscle cells, is an excellent energy source as it contains lots of chains of glucose that are readily accessible when needed. In contrast, fatty acids within your adipose (fat) cells are stored as triglycerides – three chains of fatty acids each bound to a molecule of glycerol – that take longer to break down and burn as a fuel.

As each of the twenty-one amino acids vary in structure, the body uses twenty-one different metabolic pathways to process them and release substances that your body can use to produce energy. When following a balanced diet, these pathways normally account for between 10 and 15 per cent of the energy your body produces. When you follow a high-protein diet, however, the amount of energy derived from dietary proteins increases, and your liver produces more of the enzymes needed to process them as an efficient energy source.

Dietary carbohydrates

Carbohydrates are usually the main energy source within your diet. As your body can make all the various carbohydrates it needs from other sources, no dietary carbohydrates are deemed 'essential' in the same way as some amino acids and the essential fatty acids are. But as glucose is the only type of fuel that brain cells can use, it is vital that your body continues to maintain a steady blood glucose level – if dietary carbohydrates are in short supply, your liver must make glucose from other substances, especially protein.

The simplest forms of dietary carbohydrate are single sugars, or monosaccharides, such as glucose (grape sugar, also known as dextrose), galactose (a milk sugar) and fructose (a fruit sugar). Two single sugars can join together to form a double sugar (disaccharide) such as ordinary table sugar (sucrose), lactose (a milk sugar) and maltose (a sugar found in cereals). Sugar molecules can also form chains. Those formed from three to ten sugars are known as oligosaccharides. Those containing a greater number of conjoined sugars, such as starch, are called polysaccharides.

The types of carbohydrate in your diet are shown in Table 1.

Table 1 Simple and complex dietary carbohydrates

Types of carbohydrate	Examples
Monosaccharides	glucose (grape sugar) galactose (a milk sugar) fructose (fruit sugar) deoxyribose (a sugar used to make your DNA)
Disaccharides	sucrose (glucose + fructose) lactose (glucose + galactose) maltose (glucose + glucose)
Oligosaccharides	fructo-oligosaccharides (short chains of fructose) galacto-oligosaccharides (short chains of galactose)
Polysaccharides	starch, glycogen, inulin, cellulose

Simple sugars (monosaccharides) pass from your intestines into your bloodstream unchanged. Because disaccharides are made up of two sugar molecules joined together, they must first be separated into their individual monosaccharides by digestive enzymes (salivary and pancreatic amylase) before they are absorbed. The digestion of starch takes even longer, but releases a steady stream of simpler sugars into the circulation, which helps to maintain an even blood-glucose level. Many plant oligosaccharides and polysaccharides, however, cannot be broken down as our bodies lack the enzymes needed to digest them. Instead these form the bulk of dietary fibre – a crucial dietary component which is explored later.

Monosaccharides pass through the gut wall into your circulation and travel directly to your liver via the hepatic portal vein. Most are taken up by your liver cells, as one of their most important jobs is to maintain blood sugar levels by releasing a constant supply of glucose. When dietary glucose is plentiful, excess is stored as glycogen, a starchy emergency fuel, or converted into fat for long-term energy storage. When dietary glucose is in short supply, the liver can also make new glucose from fructose, glycerol, lactic acid and certain amino acids – but not from fatty acids. In fact, the conversion of milk and meat proteins to glucose is so efficient that your liver can produce 50 g of glucose from 100 g of protein.

Glucose is an important fuel for all your body cells, but different cells absorb it with different degrees of efficiency. Liver and brain cells contain special proteins that act like pores to allow glucose free entry into these cells. However, muscle and adipose (fat) cells contain a different type of glucose receptor known as Glut-4 glucose transporters, which only allow glucose to enter the cell if the hormone insulin is present. This is because Glut-4 transporters are stored *inside* the cells and only come to the surface to provide a glucose entry channel when insulin is present.

When insulin levels fall, the Glut-4 transporter proteins move back into the centre of the cell, closing the channel so that glucose can no longer enter. This mechanism is thought to ensure that some glucose remains in your circulation at all times, for use by your brain cells, for which glucose is such a vital fuel that they can absorb it without the need for insulin.

Insulin is made in your pancreas, a gland that lies just beneath the stomach. The pancreas contains millions of clusters of specialized cells (the Islets of Langerhans) that secrete a variety of digestive enzymes and hormones. The scientists who first discovered these named the types of cell according to the first letters of the Greek alphabet, and it is now known that it is the beta cells that secrete insulin in response to a rise in your blood glucose concentrations. This increase in insulin production occurs within minutes of glucose levels rising after a meal, and provides the key to start letting glucose into muscle and fat cells. Once inside muscle cells, glucose is burned to produce energy, and excess is converted into glycogen. Within fat (adipose) cells, excess glucose is converted into triglyceride fats for storage, as we will discuss shortly.

As glucose moves out of the circulation, and blood glucose levels fall, the beta cells stop producing insulin. Glut-4 transporter proteins move back into the centre of muscle and fat cells so glucose can no longer enter. If blood glucose levels fall too low, another type of pancreatic cell – this time the alpha cells – secrete another hormone, glucagon, which has the opposite effect to insulin. Glucagon causes the liver to break down its glycogen stores to release glucose back into the circulation. In this way, circulating blood glucose levels are normally kept within a tight range. Different units of measurement are used in different parts of the world, so a normal glucose range is either 3.9 to 5.6 mmol/l (millimoles per litre) in the UK, or 70 to 100 mg/dl (milligrams per decilitre) in the US.

Both the type and amount of carbohydrate in your diet has a major impact on your blood glucose levels and your secretion of insulin and glucagon. Glucose causes a rapid rise in blood glucose levels, while other simple sugars (monosaccharides), such as fructose and galactose, have a lesser effect as it takes time for the liver to convert them into glucose. Starch releases a steady stream of glucose to produce a lower, but more sustained rise in blood glucose levels.

Glycaemic Index

The way in which different carbohydrates affect your blood glucose levels can be measured and quantified. This concept, known as the Glycaemic Index (GI), rates how eating 50 g of digestible carbohydrate from different foods affects your blood glucose levels, compared with eating the same amount of glucose. The effect of glucose is given an arbitrary GI value of 100, so a food

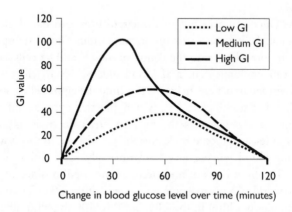

Diagram 1 Relationship between a food's Glycaemic Index and blood glucose levels

that raises blood glucose levels by half as much is assigned a GI value of 50.

Foods with a high GI (70 or above) have a rapid effect on your blood glucose levels (see solid line on the graph above). Foods with a medium GI (56 to 69) have a more sustained effect on your blood glucose levels (see dashed line on the graph above), while foods with a low GI (less than 55, see dotted line on the graph above) contain few carbohydrates, or carbohydrates that are metabolized slowly and have only a minor effect on your blood glucose levels.

Although the Glycaemic Index is a useful concept to help you select a healthy diet, it is based on eating whatever quantity of food contains 50 g of digestible carbohydrate. In the case of parsnips, for example, a steep rise in blood glucose levels would only occur after eating more than most people could manage, and you don't need to worry about including them in your diet. Similarly, an average serving of white pasta contains considerably more than 50 g digestible carbohydrate and has a larger impact on your blood glucose levels than you might expect from its GI alone.

Hence another, more realistic system has been developed called the Glycaemic Load (GL). This provides more useful information, as it takes into account the amount of carbohydrate present in a typical portion.

GLYCAEMIC LOAD (GL)

The GL of a food is calculated by multiplying that food's GI value by the amount of carbohydrate measured in grams found in a typical serving, then dividing the result by 100 as a percentage.

Foods classed as having a high GL (20 or more) release energy quickly, within minutes. Those with a low GL (10 or less) are digested, absorbed and processed to release glucose more slowly, over several hours. Those with a medium GL (11 to 19) have a moderate effect on your blood glucose levels.

Some useful GL values are given in Table 2.

After eating a carbohydrate–rich meal, the rate at which blood glucose levels rise to trigger an insulin response depends on the balance of monosaccharides, disaccharides and complex carbohydrates you have eaten. Monosaccharides cause a rapid rise, disaccharides a moderate rise and complex carbohydrates a lesser but more prolonged response. It also depends on the amount of fibre and fat present in the meal, as these help to slow the digestion and absorption of carbohydrates. For example, eating bread and butter produces a slower rise in blood glucose levels than eating a slice of bread alone.

Table 2 GI and GL values for popular foods

Foods with a high GL	Foods with a medium GL	Foods with a low GL
White rice, boiled	Cornflakes	Muesli
Condensed milk	Wholemeal spaghetti, boiled	Sweetcorn, boiled
Raisins	Dried, tenderized figs	Dried apricots
Baked potato, without skin	Brown rice, steamed	Wholemeal rye bread
White spaghetti, boiled	New potatoes, boiled	Most fresh fruit and vegetables
	Banana, ripe	Cooked beans
	Unsweetened fruit juices	Parsnips, boiled
	Honey	Carrots
	Oat porridge	
	Sweet potato	
	White bread	

GI and GL values vary slightly from different sources. A large searchable database is available, free, at a University of Sydney website: www.glycemicindex.com

POLYOLS

Some 'diet' products contain sugar-free sweeteners such as xylitol, lactitol, sorbitol and maltitol. These polyols are classed as carbohydrates as they are derived from sugars, but despite their sweet taste, they are not processed in the body like sugars and do not promote tooth decay. Sorbitol, lactitol and xylitol do not raise blood glucose levels, but maltitol has the same effect on blood glucose levels as sucrose. In practice, however, the consumption of polyols is limited by their laxative effect. Some people are more sensitive to this than others, so that intakes above 10 g to 20 g per day can cause flatulence, bloating and diarrhoea.

Dietary fibre

Dietary fibre – sometimes referred to as 'roughage' – consists of the non-digestible carbohydrates in your diet. While fibre passes through your small intestines unchanged, and provides little in the way of energy or nutrients, it encourages peristalsis and aids the digestion and absorption of other foods.

There are two main types: soluble and insoluble fibre. All plant foods contain both types, but some sources are richer in one type than another. Oats, figs, barley, apples, prunes and kidney beans, for example, are rich in soluble fibre, while wheat, brown rice, rhubarb, leafy vegetables, peas and chickpeas are good sources of insoluble fibre.

Soluble fibre (such as pectins, gums and mucilage) form a gel when mixed with liquid and is particularly important in the stomach and upper intestines. It slows the digestion and absorption of other carbohydrates, helping to blunt the rate at which blood glucose levels rise. It also attracts fats to slow their absorption, and lowers blood fat levels. Once soluble fibre reaches the large bowel, it is fermented by bacterial enzymes to release nutrients and smelly gases. Insoluble fibre (e.g. cellulose) is most important in the large bowel, where it adds bulk, absorbs water, bacteria and toxins and hastens stool excretion. Much of the increased bulk of bowel motions associated with a high-fibre diet is due to increased bacterial multiplication in the gut. For every gram of fibre eaten, bowel motions increase by around 5 g in weight.

Fibre is found mainly in fruit, vegetables and wholegrain products. Our ancestors followed a diet that provided 100 g or more of fibre per day. Ideally, you need a fibre intake of at least 20 g to 30 g daily. When increasing fibre intake, it is also important to drink at least two to three litres of fluids per day as this is absorbed by the fibre and helps to bulk it up for optimum effect.

The fibre content of various fruits and vegetables is shown in Table 3.

Table 3 Fibre content of various plant-based foods

Food	Fibre content per 100 g
Bran	36 g
Bran cereal	13 g to 25 g
Apricots, dried	18 g
Prunes	13 g
Figs, dried	8 g
Muesli (unsweetened)	8 g
Oatmeal	7 g
Kidney beans, boiled	7 g
Wholemeal bread	7 g
Mixed nuts	6 g
Peas	5 g
Dates, dried	4 g

(*Continued*)

Table 3 Cont'd

Food	Fibre content per 100 g
Wholemeal spaghetti, cooked	4 g
Brown bread	4 g
White bread	2 g
Apples, raw	2 g
Rhubarb	2 g
Pears	2 g
Brown rice, boiled	1 g

Dietary fats

Fats are the most energy-dense food groups, supplying 9 kcal energy per gram of fat (compared with 4 kcal per gram for protein and carbohydrate). It is therefore an efficient way for your body to bank excess calories for use in future lean times.

Despite their bad name, dietary fats are vital for good nutrition. Like protein, fatty acids play an important structural role in the body, providing building blocks for making cell membranes and nerve sheaths. They are also used to make sex hormones, immune regulators and bile salts and to transport fat-soluble nutrients such as vitamins A, D, E and K. However, eating too much fat is associated with weight gain and can have adverse effects on blood fat levels and your risk of coronary heart disease. Current advice is that dietary fats should provide no more than 30 per cent of daily energy intake. For someone with an average energy intake of 2,000 kcal per day, 30 per cent of energy intake represents around 67 g of fat (1 g fat supplies 9 kcals energy).

The basic building blocks of fat are called free fatty acids (carboxylic acids). These contain a chain of carbon atoms that are linked to each other through single or double chemical bonds.

A fatty acid whose carbon atoms are joined using only single bonds is described as saturated, as all its available bonds are fully saturated with additional hydrogen atoms. A fatty acid that contains one or more double bonds is known as an unsaturated fat; of these, a fatty acid with a single double chemical bond is described as monounsaturated, while one with two or more double bonds is referred to as polyunsaturated.

The number and position of the double bonds within a fatty acid determines whether it acts as a solid or liquid at room temperature. In general, saturated fats tend to be solid at room temperature, while monounsaturated and polyunsaturated fats tend to be oils. The position of the double bonds also determines how the fatty acid is metabolized in your body.

Triglycerides

The fats in your diet, and in your body stores, are mainly in the form of triglycerides. These E-shaped molecules contain three fatty-acid chains linked to a glycerol backbone. The three fatty-acid chains in a triglyceride molecule do not have to be the same. One could be a saturated fatty acid, one a monounsaturated fatty acid and one a polyunsaturated fatty acid. Most fats contain a blend of these three different types of fatty acids. Almost half (47 per cent) of the fatty acids found in beef fat are monounsaturated, for example, even though this animal fat is classed as saturated.

In general, animal-based foods contain a higher percentage of saturated fat than vegetable foods. The exact breakdown will vary depending on the country, and how the animals or plants from which the fats are obtained were farmed. For example, grass-fed cattle tend to have a healthier fatty-acid composition, with more essential fatty acids, omega-3 polyunsaturated fats and antioxidants than grain-fed cattle. The fat from grass-fed beef may also have a more yellow appearance due to the higher content of beneficial carotenoid pigments. This is especially true of Guernsey

Channel Island cows, whose fat (and the butter and cream made from their milk) is a lovely rich colour. Why? Because these cattle are genetically less efficient at converting the yellow carotenoid pigment, betacarotene, on to vitamin A. Despite these considerations, typical values for the types of fatty acid obtained from a variety of sources are shown in Table 4. Those with the least saturated fat and the most monounsaturated fat are usually considered the most healthy, which is why nutritionists encourage you to use more olive, nut and rapeseed oils during cooking and in salad dressings, rather than corn and safflower oils.

Table 4 Typical fatty-acid composition of various dietary fats

Dietary fat	% saturated	% polyunsaturated	% monounsaturated
Macadamia nut oil	14%	5%	81%
Hazelnut oil	8%	14%	78%
Olive oil	15%	10%	75%
Almond oil	8%	18%	74%
Rapeseed oil	7%	32%	61%
Walnut oil	10%	70%	20%
Flaxseed oil	9%	72%	19%
Safflower oil	10%	76%	14%
Sunflower oil	12%	22%	66%
Corn oil	13%	58%	29%
Beef fat (dripping)	50%	3%	47%
Pork fat (lard)	43%	10%	47%
Butter fat	68%	4%	28%

Saturated fats

Saturated fats have gained a reputation as 'bad' fats, as consuming an excess of these has been associated with an increased risk of coronary heart disease. Not all studies show this, however, and, although it is commonly believed that saturated fats are converted into cholesterol in the liver, this is not absolutely true. Only saturated fatty acids with chain lengths of 12, 14 or 16 carbon atoms have an effect on your blood cholesterol levels. Saturated fats with other chain lengths are not converted into cholesterol in the liver at all, and therefore have a neutral effect on your cholesterol levels. Overall, a third of dietary saturated fats – including stearic acid (18 carbon atoms) found in milk fat, cocoa butter and meat fat – have no cholesterol-raising activity. This does not mean that a high saturated-fat intake is harmless. Like all types of fat, it has a high calorie content and an excess is linked with obesity. And, if you have a high cholesterol level, you may have inherited genes that mean you process saturated fat less efficiently than other people. Ideally, saturated fats should supply no more than 7 to ten 10 cent of your energy intake, which, for most people, means cutting back. Replace them with more beneficial mono-unsaturated fatty acids (found in olive, rapeseed, macadamia and avocado or walnut oils, as shown in Table 4), or omega-3 polyun-saturated fats (found in fish, flaxseed and walnuts oils).

Monounsaturated fats

Monounsaturated fats, such as oleic acid, consist of chains of carbon atoms in which there is only one double (unsaturated) bond. They are metabolized in such a way that they lower blood levels of harmful low-density-lipoprotein (LDL) cholesterol but have no effect on beneficial high-density-lipoprotein (HDL) cholesterol. As such, a diet high in monounsaturates may help to reduce your risk of atherosclerosis, high blood pressure, coronary heart disease and stroke. This is thought to explain some of the benefits of the so-called Mediterranean diet. Ideally, monounsaturated fats should supply around 12 per cent of your energy intake. For most people, this means eating more monounsaturates.

Polyunsaturated fats

Polyunsaturated fatty acids (PUFAs) have a molecular structure whose carbon chains contain two or more double bonds. There are two main types of polyunsaturated fat in the diet: if the *first* double bond involves the third carbon atom, it is classed as an omega-3 fatty acid; if the *first* double bond involves the sixth carbon atom, it is classed as an omega-6 fatty acid.

PEROXIDES

Having so many double bonds makes polyunsaturated fats highly reactive and susceptible to chemical changes known as oxidation. This can produce toxic substances (lipid peroxides) that are believed to trigger hardening and furring-up of artery walls if there are insufficient antioxidants to prevent oxidation. Factors which encourage the formation of these toxic lipid peroxides include eating excessive amounts of polyunsaturated fats (PUFAs), over-heating PUFA oils so they smoke while cooking and reheating cooking oils.

Because of the position of their first double bond, your body handles omega-3 and omega-6 oils in different ways. Omega-6 fatty acids are converted into substances (series 2 prostaglandins, series 4 leukotrienes) that tend to have an inflammatory action and increase blood stickiness, which can lead to unwanted blood clots. In contrast, omega-3 fatty acids act as building blocks to make substances (series 3 prostaglandins, series 5 leukotrienes) that are anti-inflammatory and have a blood-thinning action.

The omega-6 fatty acid, gamma-linolenic acid (GLA) is one of the few omega-6s that can reduce inflammation if intake is sufficiently high. It is found in evening primrose and starflower oils, which are popular supplements for people with dry, itchy skin such as in eczema (an inflammatory condition).

Essential fatty acids

You cannot make the short-chain omega-6, linoleic acid, or the short-chain omega-3, alpha-linolenic acid. These two fatty acids are therefore classed as 'essential', as they must come from your diet. Ideally, linoleic acid should supply at least 1 per cent of your energy intake, and linolenic acid at least 0.2 per cent. Once you consume these 'parent' polyunsaturates, however, your body can convert them on to longer-chain PUFAs (such as DHA and EPA) which are important for healthy brain and eye function. However, omega-6 fatty acids cannot be converted into omega-3 fatty acids in the body, or vice versa. Linoleic acid can only be converted into other omega-6 fatty acids, such as gamma-linolenic acid (GLA) and arachidonic acid (AA), while alpha-linolenic acid can only be converted on to other omega-3 fatty acids such as eicosapentaenoic acid (EPA) and docosahexaenoic acid (DHA). The way your body makes these longer-chain polyunsaturated fatty acids involves two important metabolic pathways, as shown in Diagram 2.

This method of lengthening the parent short-chain essential fatty acids (LA and ALA) as shown in Diagram 2 is not that efficient, and the enzymes involved are readily blocked by a number of factors associated with an unhealthy diet, lifestyle and toxicity, including excess intakes of saturated fats, trans-fatty acids, sugar or alcohol; dietary lack of vitamins and minerals, especially vitamin B6, zinc and magnesium; crash-dieting; smoking cigarettes and exposure to pollution.

As a result, only around 5 per cent of dietary alpha-linolenic acid (ALA) is converted on to the important long-chain omega-3

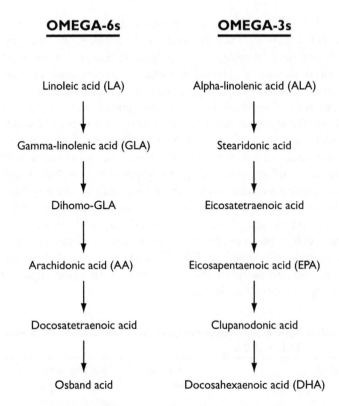

OMEGA-6s	OMEGA-3s
Linoleic acid (LA)	Alpha-linolenic acid (ALA)
↓	↓
Gamma-linolenic acid (GLA)	Stearidonic acid
↓	↓
Dihomo-GLA	Eicosatetraenoic acid
↓	↓
Arachidonic acid (AA)	Eicosapentaenoic acid (EPA)
↓	↓
Docosatetraenoic acid	Clupanodonic acid
↓	↓
Osband acid	Docosahexaenoic acid (DHA)

Diagram 2 Synthesis of long-chain PUFAs from short-chain essential fatty acids

polyunsaturated fatty acid EPA, and only 0.5 per cent is further converted on to form DHA. These long-chain fatty acids are therefore often classed as essential, too.

The long-chain polyunsaturated fatty acids are also important for good nutrition. They act as building blocks for making the membranes found in all body cells, including heart muscle cells, brain cells and artery lining cells. The long-chain omega-3s, DHA and EPA, are especially important for healthy brain and eye function.

A healthy adult needs to consume around 6 g to 10 g of essential fatty acids per day, in the right balance. Our ancestors evolved on a Stone Age diet supplying an omega-6 to omega-3 ratio of around 2:1. The average Western diet currently contains a ratio of omega-6 to omega-3 fats of 10:1 due to increased consumption of vegetable oils, vegetables spreads and convenience foods. We also tend to eat fewer omega-3 rich nuts and less oily fish than in the past. Most people would benefit from increasing their intake of anti-inflammatory omega-3s, and reducing their intake of inflammatory omega-6s, which have been linked with inflammatory diseases such as asthma, eczema and coronary heart disease (which is now recognized as an inflammatory process).

Good sources of omega-3 essential fatty acids include: oily fish such as mackerel, herring, salmon, trout, sardines, pilchards, fresh tuna (not tinned, see Table 5); wild game meat such as venison and buffalo; grass-fed beef; omega-3 enriched eggs; and omega-3 fish-oil supplements.

Table 5 Typical long-chain omega-3 fatty-acid content (EPA plus DHA) of fish

Food	Portion size (grams)	Total long-chain omega-3s per portion (grams)
Kippers	150 g	3.89 g
Salmon	150 g	3.25 g
Mackerel	150 g	2.89 g
Pilchards (in tomato sauce)	110 g	2.86 g
Herring	150 g	1.97 g
Tuna (fresh)	150 g	1.95 g
Trout	150 g	1.73 g

(*Continued*)

Table 5 Cont'd

Food	Portion size (grams)	Total long-chain omega-3s per portion (grams)
Sardines (in tomato sauce)	100 g	1.67 g
Salmon (canned in brine)	100 g	1.55 g
Plaice	150 g	0.45 g
Cod	150 g	0.38 g
Haddock	150 g	0.24 g
Tuna (in oil, drained)	45 g	0.17 g
Tuna (in brine, drained)	45 g	0.08 g

You can reduce your intake of inflammatory omega-6s by consuming fewer omega-6-rich vegetable oils such as safflower oil, grapeseed oil, sunflower oil, corn oil, cottonseed oil or soybean oil (replace with healthier oils such as rapeseed, olive or walnut oils); margarines based on omega-6 oils such as sunflower or safflower oil; convenience foods; fast foods; manufactured goods such as cakes, sweets and pastries.

Essential fatty-acid deficiency

When you do not get enough essential fatty acids (EFAs) in your diet, your body makes do with the next-best fatty acids available. It incorporates saturated fatty acids and even harmful trans-fatty acids into cell membranes. These fatty acids have a less flexible structure, however, and may affect the elasticity of your arteries, and the speed at which chemical and electrical messages are passed within your nervous system.

Lack of omega-3 essential fatty acids during infancy and childhood has been linked to an increased risk of allergies such as eczema, asthma and hay fever. It has also been associated with learning difficulties such as dyslexia. Symptoms that may be due to an essential fatty-acid deficiency are:

- excessive thirst
- frequent urination
- dry, scaly, itchy skin
- keratosis pilaris (pimply 'goosebump' skin on the upper arms and legs)
- dull, straw-like hair and soft or brittle nails
- impaired immunity, with frequent infections
- atopic conditions (eczema, hayfever, asthma)
- visual difficulties (poor night vision, sensitivity to bright light, visual disturbances when reading)
- learning difficulties (distractibility, poor concentration, poor working memory)
- emotional sensitivity (depression, excessive mood swings, undue anxiety)
- sleep problems (difficulty settling at night, early waking).

Trans-fatty acids

Polyunsaturated fatty acids are oils at room temperature. They can be converted into semi-solid margarines and spreads by incorporating extra hydrogen atoms into their chemical structure to convert some double bonds to single bonds. Some of these artificially produced, partially hydrogenated fats have a twisted structure and are known as trans-fatty acids.

The body processes trans-fats in a way that is harmful to health. They increase the rigidity of your cell membranes, raise blood levels of 'bad' LDL-cholesterol, lower 'good' HDL cholesterol, increase inflammation and may also affect glucose control and promote weight gain. They may also block the metabolism of essential fatty acids so that their beneficial effects are not fully realized. As if this weren't enough, trans-fats were recently also linked with the development of certain cancers, especially of the breast and prostate gland. As a result, margarines and low-fat spreads are now being reformulated to reduce their trans-fat content. Some countries have introduced guidelines aimed at reducing intakes of trans-fatty acids to no more than 2 per cent of your total energy intake. Always check labels and select foods with the lowest content of trans-fats or partially hydrogenated polyunsaturated fats.

NATURAL VS ARTIFICIAL

Natural trans-fatty acids are produced in the rumen of cattle, sheep and goats. Small amounts of trans-fats (2 to 4 per cent) are therefore found in milk, cheese, butter and meat. These naturally occurring trans-fats are structurally different from those produced commercially during the hydrogenation of fats, however, and have not been implicated in increasing health risks such as coronary heart disease. This has turned the butter-versus-margarine controversy on its head, as some scientists now believe it is healthier to eat butter than margarine or low-fat spreads. The simplest advice is to eat as wide a variety of foods as possible, including a little of everything (butter and margarine, if you wish) and to eat nothing to excess.

Cholesterol

Cholesterol is a fatty substance made in animal livers. Your own liver makes around 800 mg cholesterol every day from certain fats in your diet. You also obtain some – around 300 mg per day – from animal-based foods such as meat, egg yolks and prawns (see Table 6).

Table 6 Cholesterol content of common foods

Food	Cholesterol content per 100 g
Pig's liver	700 mg
Lamb's kidney	610 mg
Caviar	588 mg
Lamb's liver	400 mg
Chicken liver	350 mg
Calf's liver	330 mg
Prawns	280 mg
Pheasant meat	220 mg
Butter	213 mg
Squid	200 mg
Duck meat	110 mg
Lobster meat	110 mg
Chicken meat (dark)	105 mg
Hard cheese	100 mg
Lean beef	58 mg
Chicken meat (white)	70 mg

Although cholesterol has a bad name, a certain amount is vital for health. Like other fats, it acts as an important building block to make healthy cell membranes, steroid hormones (e.g. cortisol, oestrogen, testosterone, progesterone), vitamin D, bile acids and coenzyme Q10 – a vitamin-like substance essential for processing oxygen and generating energy within cells.

If you make or eat too much cholesterol, however, your risk of coronary heart disease may increase through a process known as atherosclerosis.

ATHEROSCLEROSIS

If you lack dietary antioxidants (found in fruit and vegetables) the cholesterol in your circulation undergoes a chemical reaction called oxidation. Immune scavenger cells (macrophages) do not recognize the oxidized cholesterol and absorb it in an attempt to remove 'foreign' material from your circulation. If circulating levels are high, they soon form bloated 'foam' cells. When they try to leave your bloodstream by squeezing through cells in your artery linings, they become trapped and contribute to hardening and furring-up of the arteries (atherosclerosis).

As cholesterol is insoluble, your liver packages it with special proteins to make it soluble before releasing it into your circulation. These proteins surround the cholesterol to form spherical particles known as lipoproteins. Insoluble cholesterol stays on the inside, and the proteins, which have an affinity for both fat and water, remain on the outside.

Low-density lipoprotein (LDL) cholesterol forms small, light particles that can seep into your artery walls. LDL-cholesterol is also prone to oxidation and is readily engulfed by scavenger cells. The higher your level of LDL-cholesterol, the higher your risk of atherosclerosis and cardiovascular disease.

High-density lipoprotein (HDL) cholesterol forms larger, heavier particles that are too big to seep into artery walls. For every 1 per cent rise in your blood level of HDL-cholesterol, your risk of cardiovascular disease falls by as much as 2 per cent. This is due to reversed cholesterol transport in which HDL sweeps excess LDL-cholesterol away from your circulation and carries it back to your liver for processing.

CHOLESTEROL BALANCE

Your blood cholesterol level is a balance between the amount of cholesterol released into your circulation by your liver, and the amount removed from your circulation by body cells. When a cell needs cholesterol it sends LDL-receptors to its surface to 'catch' passing LDL particles. Most (70 per cent) of the cholesterol removed from your circulation is taken back up by liver cells and usually suppresses their need to produce new cholesterol. Some people inherit genes that are less sensitive to this suppression so that their liver produces more and more cholesterol, even though their levels are adequate. Others have faulty LDL-receptors that are less efficient at trapping and absorbing circulating cholesterol, so LDL-particles remain in the circulation for longer than the normal average of two and a half days.

The optimal level for cholesterol is not clear-cut but in general you want:

- a total cholesterol of less than 5 mmol/l (200 mg/dl)
- an LDL-cholesterol of less than 3 mmol/l (100 mg/dl)
- an HDL-cholesterol greater than 1 mmol/l (40 mg/dl) for men, or 1.2 mmol/l (50 mg/dl) for women.

If you have other risk factors for cardiovascular disease (e.g. smoking, high blood pressure, diabetes) the recommended total cholesterol level is even lower (below 4 mmol/l) with an LDL-cholesterol of less than 2 mmol/l. Because this is difficult to achieve via diet, it usually means taking a statin drug.

Low-cholesterol diet

Dietary changes can lower your total and 'bad' LDL–cholesterol level while raising your 'good' HDL–cholesterol. Traditional advice is to lower your intake of cholesterol-rich foods (especially liver and caviar) and to cut back on saturated fats, as these are what your liver uses to make cholesterol.

Although eggs used to be frowned on, studies show that, in most people, eating eggs has minimal impact on LDL-cholesterol levels while providing health benefits in the form of antioxidants, omega-3 fatty acids and important vitamins and minerals. In fact, research involving over 100,000 men and women shows that eating one egg a day does not increase the risk of coronary heart disease or stroke – even if your cholesterol level is raised.

You may also be advised to eat more porridge oats, as many studies now show that oats, oatmeal and other oat-based products, such as porridge, can reduce 'bad' LDL-cholesterol. Why? Because oats contain fibre, which acts like a sponge to bind cholesterol and slow its absorption, and because they contain substances (betaglucans) that act on the liver to reduce your own natural cholesterol production. Similarly, snacking on a handful of almonds, walnuts or macadamia nuts per day has been shown to lower LDL-cholesterol and increase HDL-cholesterol.

STEROLS AND STANOLS

Just as animals make cholesterol, plants produce similar chemicals called sterols and stanols. These have a similar structure to human cholesterol and can block the receptors that absorb cholesterol in your small intestines without being absorbed themselves. As a result, people who eat the most plant sterols have the lowest cholesterol levels. They occur naturally in small quantities in vegetable oils, nuts, seeds, grain products, fruit and vegetables, but for optimum cholesterol-lowering benefits, you need to consume at least 2 g per day. The average diet provides less than 500 mg plant sterols/stanols daily, so foods fortified with sterols and stanols (spreads, yogurts) or sterol supplements are needed to boost intakes if you have a raised cholesterol level. Using these products can lower your LDL-cholesterol by 10 per cent within as little as 3 weeks.

3
Fuelling up: energy

Unlike plants, you cannot synthesize energy using the power of sunlight, so all the energy produced in your body must ultimately derive from the macronutrients in your diet – the proteins, carbohydrates and fatty acids.

Kilocalories and kilojoules

Energy is the dynamic force that fuels all the biological processes of life. You need energy for everything you do – from physical activities such as walking, running and playing sports, to thinking and storing memories. Energy is especially important for growth and reproduction.

The chemical energy in food can be measured in units known as calories. This is also called the standard calorie (cal) spelt with a small 'c'. The unit you are probably more familiar with, and which is used when discussing slimming diets, is the kilocalorie or kcal. This is also known as the Calorie which, by convention, is spelt with a big 'C'. One kilocalorie (kcal) is equivalent to 1,000 calories.

Because of the confusion caused between calories with a small 'c' and Calories with a big 'C', scientists now tend to use a more modern, SI unit called the joule.

Around half of your daily energy expenditure is used up through general physical activity. The other half of your energy expenditure is used up by basic metabolic functions, such as maintaining your heartbeat, respiration, digestion, body temperature and cell division. This is known as your basal metabolic rate (BMR).

ENERGY DEFINITIONS

One calorie is defined as the amount of heat energy needed to raise the temperature of 1 g of water by 1 °C from 15 °C to 16 °C.One joule is defined as the energy expended (work done) when applying a force of 1 Newton through a distance of 1 metre. Put simply, 1 joule is essentially the amount of energy needed to lift a small apple 1 metre straight up into the air.

1 kilocalorie (kcal) = 1,000 calories
1 kilojoule (kJ) = 1,000 joules
1 kcal = 4.2 kJ
1,000kj = 1 Megajoule (MJ)

Basal metabolic rate

Your BMR is tightly defined as the energy you expend just lying in bed, at complete physical and mental rest, twelve to fourteen hours after last eating, in an ambient temperature of 26 °C to 30 °C. The three main cell activities that contribute to your basal metabolic rate are:

- synthesis of chemicals in cells: proteins, fats, glucose, urea, neurotransmitters (40 per cent BMR)
- active transport of salts and proteins across cell membranes, especially the sodium–potassium pump, which forces sodium out of your cells by swapping it for potassium which is forced inside your cells; this maintains the electrical charge across your cell membranes which is vital for life (38 per cent BMR)
- involuntary muscular activity: breathing, heartbeat, gut peristalsis (22 per cent BMR).

Your basal metabolic rate varies depending on your age, gender, muscle bulk (lean body-mass percentage), nutritional status and genetic inheritance, which dictates the efficiency of metabolic reactions. The type of food you eat also plays a role as energy is used up, and heat produced, during its metabolism. This effect is known as dietary-induced thermogenesis and accounts for 10 per cent or more of the energy provided by foods.

It is possible to estimate your average BMR, based on your weight, age and gender, using mathematical formulae known as the Schofield equations (Table 7).

Table 7 Basal metabolic rate (kcal/day)

Age (years)	Males	Females
0–3	BMR = 60.9W −54	BMR = 61.0W −51
3–10	BMR = 22.7W + 495	BMR = 22.5W + 499
10–17	BMR = 17.5W + 651	BMR = 12.2W + 749
18–29	BMR = 15.3W + 679	BMR = 14.7W + 496
30–59	BMR = 11.6W + 879	BMR = 8.7W + 829
Over 60	BMR = 13.5W + 487	BMR = 10.5W + 596

BMR = basal metabolic rate; W = body weight in kilograms

For example:

A 50-year-old male weighing 70 kg has a BMR of (11.6 × 70) + 879 = 1,691 kcal/day.
A 40-year-old woman weighing 60 kg has a BMR of (8.7 × 60) + 829 = 1,351 kcal/day.

Additional energy is also needed to fuel physical activity, depending on your weight, the type of activity and its duration.

Calculating total energy requirements

The most accurate way to measure your total energy expenditure is to put you in an insulated chamber and directly measure the heat loss from your body. This is known as direct calorimetry.

Another way, known as indirect calorimetry, predicts your energy expenditure by measuring the amount of oxygen you consume, the amount of carbon dioxide (a waste gas) you exhale, and the amount of nitrogen you excrete. Together, these measurements show how much protein, carbohydrate and fat your body has burned as a fuel.

These are complex, time-consuming processes, for which volunteers are thin on the ground – few people are happy to spend a day locked in a chamber or having their body wastes closely measured and scrutinized. This being the case, scientists usually estimate energy requirements by multiplying your basal metabolic rate (BMR, predicted from the Schofield equations shown in Table 7) by a factor known as your physical activity level (PAL). The PAL takes into account all the activities you do during the day. Your total energy requirement is calculated by multiplying your BMR by your PAL.

Energy requirement = BMR × PAL

For a sedentary person who sits around all day (your average couch potato), PAL is about 1.2.

For a lightly active person (such as an office worker stuck at a desk all day), PAL works out at 1.4.

A person who is moderately active during both work and leisure activities (a sales representative, perhaps) will have a PAL of 1.6 (females) or 1.7 (males).

An individual with high levels of physical activity during both work and leisure time (a sporty type who is always on the go) has a PAL of 1.8 (females) or 1.9 (males).

Individuals with a vigorously active lifestyle, such as an elite athlete, may have a PAL of 2 to 2.4.

To work out your daily energy needs, multiply your BMR by your PAL.

In the examples above, the 50-year-old male weighing 70 kg had a BMR of 1,691 kcal/day. If he drives to and from work, has a desk job and rarely exercises in his spare time, his PAL is 1.2. His estimated total energy requirement per day is therefore: BMR (1,691) x PAL (1.2), and he needs around 2,029 kcal per day.

The 40-year-old woman who weighs 60 kg and has a BMR of 1,351 kcal/day is very active, however. She jogs to and from work, is on her feet all day and plays sport most evenings and weekends, giving her a PAL of 1.8. Her estimated total energy requirement per day is therefore: BMR (1,351) x PAL (1.8), and means she needs to eat around 2,432 kcal per day.

These types of calculations suggest that the averagely active adult male needs around 2,605 kcal (10.9 MJ) per day, while the average adult female needs around 2,079 kcal (8.7 MJ). The values vary according to age, as shown in Table 8.

Table 8 Average daily energy needs for males and females (kilocalories)

Age	Males (kcal)	Females (kcal)
0–2 months★	574	502
3–4 months★	598	550
5–6 months★	622	574
7–12 months★	718	646
1–3 years	765, 1,004, 1,171	717, 932, 1,076
4–6 years	1,386, 1,482, 1,577	1,291, 1,362, 1,482
7–10 years	1,649, 1,745, 1,840, 2,032	1,530, 1,625, 1,721, 1,936

(*Continued*)

Table 8 Cont'd

Age	Males (kcal)	Females (kcal)
11–14 years	2,127, 2,247, 2,414, 2,629	2,032, 2,103, 2,223, 2,342
15–18 years	2,820, 2,964, 3,083, 3,155	2,390, 2,414, 2,462, 2,462
19–24 years	2,772	2,175
25–34 years	2,749	2,175
35–44 years	2,629	2,103
45–54 years	2,581	2,103
55–64 years	2,581	2,079
65–74 years	2,342	1,912
Over 75 years	2,294	1,840

NB Based on UK dietary reference values for energy, updated in 2011

★ = Mixed breast/bottle feeding or unknown

A person who is maintaining their weight will have an energy intake that balances the amount of energy they expend as a result of their basal metabolic rate plus their physical activity. In general, someone who is slowly cutting back on energy intake will lose weight, while someone who consumes more food energy than they need will gain weight. If you cut back on food intake too drastically, however, your body switches to a 'survival mode' designed to improve your chances of survival during lean times. Your body's use of energy becomes more efficient and less is wasted as heat, so weight loss slows.

The energy in food

Food contains different amounts of energy depending on its chemical structure. Molecules store potential energy in the bonds holding its atoms together. Your cells harness the energy stored in these chemical bonds by breaking them down and releasing energy as one molecule is converted into another.

The three food groups known as macronutrients are the main energy sources in food:

Carbohydrate provides   4 kcal (16.8 kJ) energy per gram
Protein provides   4 kcal (16.8 kJ) energy per gram
Fat provides   9 kcal (37.8 kJ) energy per gram

Alcohol is also an important energy source for some people, providing 7 kcal (29.4 kJ) per gram – more than protein and carbohydrate, but less than fat.

How energy is released from food in the body

After carbohydrates, proteins and fats have been digested and absorbed, they are processed in a slow, complex, multi-step process that generates amazing quantities of energy sources: fatty acids, amino acids and glucose. These cell fuels are then 'burned' in tiny structures, found in almost every cell in the body, called mitochondria (single – mitochondrion). Mitochondria are the cellular equivalent of rechargeable batteries, and are found in all body cells except mature red blood cells, which have none.

CELL BATTERIES

Your mitochondria have their own double membrane and their own separate, genetic material that allows them to make the special enzymes needed to release energy from glucose and fatty acids. These enzymes act as triggers to encourage chemical reactions that would otherwise not occur, or would happen extremely slowly. Mitochondria also have their own protein-production units (ribosomes), and 'reproduce' by splitting in half (binary fission) just like bacteria. In fact, mitochondria are thought to have evolved from ancient bacteria that formed a symbiotic relationship with single-celled organisms in the primordial soup, soon after life first began on earth. The single-celled organisms benefited from gaining their own equivalent of fuel-injection engines, while the bacteria gained protection from the hostile, primordial environment outside the cell.

Mitochondria use oxygen, fatty acids and glucose to generate energy-rich storage molecules known as ATP (adenosine triphosphate). These packets of energy are then used to drive other metabolic reactions. The released energy can be converted into electrical energy (nerve conduction), into other chemical bonds or into power (contraction of muscle cells, movement of protein pores).

Most cells in your body can burn either fatty acids or glucose to generate ATP, with the exception of brain cells, which can only use glucose. Some cells such as red blood cells, kidney cells and sperm cells prefer to obtain most of their energy from the oxidation of glucose. Others, such as liver cells and exercising muscle cells, prefer to obtain most of their energy from the oxidation of free fatty acids when given the choice, as this is more energy-efficient. As soon as you start exercising, however, your muscle cells switch to using glucose, or their own stores of a starchy substance known as glycogen.

Because muscle cells need so much energy, they contain the highest concentration of mitochondria, and regular exercise can both multiply the number of mitochondria found in muscle cells and increase their size. This helps to give trained athletes increased strength and stamina as their energy reserves last longer.

Producing energy from glucose

Your cells have evolved a way to liberate the energy from glucose in a controlled way so that they do not burst into flames or explode during the process. Thankfully, stories of spontaneous combustion remain a myth as, instead, your cells break down each glucose molecule using a series of over twenty different chemical reactions, the rate of which is carefully controlled by metabolic enzymes. Many of these enzymes need help in the form of vitamins, minerals and coenzymes to work properly, which is why these micronutrients are so important for health.

The combination of glucose with oxygen (oxidation) releases energy plus two waste substances: carbon dioxide and water. Most energy is used to form energy-storage molecules (ATP) but some energy is given out as heat. The overall equation for the process, known as cell respiration, is:

Glucose + oxygen → carbon dioxide + water + energy
$$C_6H_{12}O_6 + 6\ O_2 \rightarrow 6\ CO_2 + 6\ H_2O + \text{energy}$$

The breakdown of glucose to release its energy involves three different, but closely linked, metabolic pathways: glycolysis, the citric acid (Krebs) cycle and the electron transport chain.

Glycolysis

Glycolysis occurs inside the cell fluid (cytoplasm) rather than in the mitochondria. It consists of a series of nine steps that produce two molecules of an end substance called pyruvate from every molecule of glucose (see Diagram 3). Pyruvate is a useful intermediary as it can be converted back into glucose, used to make fatty acids (for storage) and used to make an amino acid (alanine). More usually, however, it is converted on to acetyl-coenzyme A then fed into the next stage of the energy-making process known as the citric acid cycle.

As you can see, glycolysis initially requires an investment of two molecules of ATP for each molecule of glucose to form an intermediary sugar (dihydroxyacetone phosphate). Once this

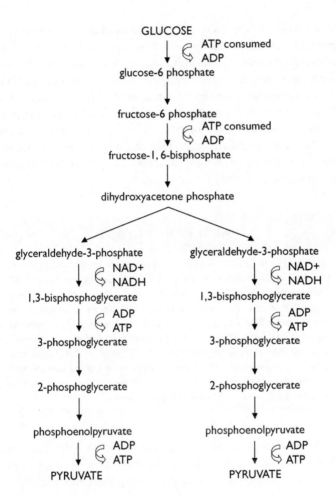

Diagram 3 Chemical steps involved in glycolysis

sugar splits in half, however, each of the two halves generates two molecules of ATP as it is converted on to pyruvate, for a net gain of two ATP molecules. In addition, each half generates a hydrogen atom, which is absorbed by a special carrier molecule, NAD+ (nicotinamide adenine dinucleotide, derived from vitamin B3). This carrier feeds the hydrogen atom into the electron transport chain – to be discussed shortly – where it is processed to release another three molecules of ATP. In this way, one glucose molecule generates a total of eight packets of energy (ATP) during the initial glycolysis pathway.

PACKETS OF ENERGY

Each molecule of ATP contains two phosphate bonds which, when 'broken' or hydrolyzed, release energy for use in the body. ATP (adenosine triphosphate) readily releases its potential energy, in a controllable amount, when a phosphate molecule splits off to leave ADP (adenosine diphosphate). ADP is then usually converted straight back into ATP again, for the next round of energy-producing reactions. It is this regeneration of ATP for which fatty acids and glucose are essential. The reactions involved in energy storage and production are collectively known as cell respiration, and result in the production of carbon dioxide plus water.

Meanwhile, back in the glycolysis pathway, the next step depends on whether oxygen is readily available (for example, when walking gently), or in short supply (during vigorous exercise).

Anaerobic glycolysis

If oxygen is in short supply, pyruvate is processed to yield its remaining energy via a rapid process known as anaerobic glycolysis, or fermentation. This also occurs in the cell cytoplasm, and involves the simple conversion of pyruvate to lactic acid (also known as lactate). This quickly generates two packets of energy (ATP) from each molecule of glucose released from a muscle's emergency stores of glycogen.

Although anaerobic fermentation provides energy at a fast rate, it is inefficient and produces much less energy than when oxygen is available. Muscle cells therefore only use anaerobic glycolysis when they absolutely have to, for example during vigorous exercise.

Interestingly, this process of anaerobic fermentation is thought to be one of the most ancient pathways in our metabolism, as life originally evolved in an atmosphere that lacked oxygen.

A COMMON CAUSE OF CRAMP

Lactic acid formed during this anaerobic fermentation enters the bloodstream and travels to the liver, where it is recycled back to glucose using oxygen. The need for extra oxygen to regenerate glucose in this way – known as the oxygen debt – is what makes you out of breath and gasping for air after brisk exercise. A build-up of lactic acid in exercising muscles can also trigger cramps. A 'stitch', for example, may involve cramping of muscle in the diaphragm, although this is controversial – a more recent idea is that a stitch is due to irritation of the peritoneal membrane lining the abdominal cavity.

When oxygen becomes plentiful again (for example, during your recovery period from exercise) muscle cells revert to the more efficient process of burning glucose with oxygen. To do this, a carrier takes pyruvate molecules from the cell fluid into the cells' energy production factories, the mitochondria. Here, pyruvate is converted into another key substance, acetyl-coenzyme A. Remember these names – pyruvate and acetyl-coenzyme

A – they are key molecules formed from the breakdown of fatty acids and protein, as well as from the breakdown of glucose.

Citric acid cycle

The citric acid cycle is arguably the most important series of metabolic reactions in your body. It is sometimes referred to as the tricarboxylic acid cycle, or the Krebs cycle, after the biochemist Sir Hans Adolf Krebs, who, in 1953, shared a Nobel Prize for its elucidation. This series of reactions takes place within the mitochondria of nearly all of your body cells.

Essentially, this cycle of chemical reactions takes acetyl-coenzyme A (formed from the breakdown of carbohydrates, fat and protein) and releases the energy contained within its chemical bonds by oxidizing it completely to form carbon dioxide and water. All the macronutrients you eat – fats, proteins and carbohydrates – can be used to make energy via this route.

Briefly, it combines acetyl-coenzyme A with another substance, oxaloacetate, to make citric acid. Citric acid then goes through a series of eight chemical reactions which convert it back into oxaloacetate, to complete one turn of the cycle (see Diagram 4).

During the citric acid cycle (in a similar process to glycolysis), hydrogen ions are released and passed to special carriers, NAD+ and FAD+ (flavine adenine dinucleotide, derived from vitamin B2) to form NADH and $FADH_2$. These carriers take the hydrogen to the next metabolic pathway, the electron transport chain, which also takes place within the mitochondria.

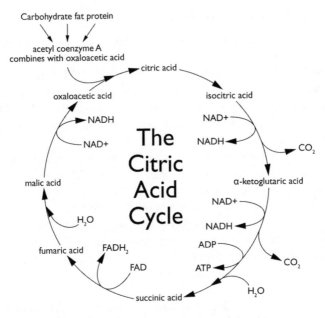

Diagram 4 Chemical steps involved in the citric acid cycle

THE CITRIC ACID CYCLE AS A SOURCE OF BUILDING BLOCKS

As well as being involved in energy production, the chemicals involved in the citric acid cycle can leave, when needed, to act as building blocks for the production of fatty acids, sterols, amino acids, haem (needed to make the red blood pigment haemoglobin), purines and pyrimidines (needed to make genetic material) and glucose. The citric acid cycle is therefore known as an amphibolic pathway, as it can be used both to break down body chemicals (catabolism) and to build them up (anabolism).

The electron transport chain

The electron transport chain acts rather like a turbo-charged, fuel-injection system, using the energy within the NADH and $FADH_2$ molecules to drive the production of ATP from ADP. Three molecules of ATP are formed from the processing of each molecule of NADH, and two from each molecule of $FADH_2$. The freed hydrogen is ultimately combined with oxygen to produce water.

The latest research suggests that the breakdown of 1 molecule of glucose ultimately yields 31 molecules of ATP via these three routes: glycolysis, the citric acid cycle and the electron transport chain (previously the value was thought to be 38).

That, in a nutshell, explains what happens when your cells 'burn' glucose to produce energy plus waste carbon dioxide gas and water. A more complete version of our earlier simplified equation for cell respiration is therefore:

Glucose + oxygen → carbon dioxide + water + 31 ATP (energy)
$C_6H_{12}O_6 + 6\ O_2$ → $6\ CO_2 + 6\ H_2O + 31$ ATP (energy)

Producing energy from dietary proteins

Dietary proteins (and, during starvation, the body's own muscle proteins) are also used to provide energy. When you are well fed, dietary proteins may first be converted to glycogen or to triglycerides for fuel storage.

To release energy from amino acids, they are first stripped of their 'amino' groups and converted into substances known as alpha-keto acids. Some of these amino groups are used to produce new amino acids (e.g. glutamine), or genetic material (nucleotides) but most are sent to the liver and made into urea, which is then excreted via the kidneys.

The alpha-keto acid part of each amino acid then enters a specific chemical pathway (one for each of the different amino acids) to form an end product (pyruvate, acetyl-coenzyme A, succinate, oxaloacetate or fumarate) that can feed into the citric acid cycle.

Once entered into the citric acid cycle, they are either oxidized to carbon dioxide and water, or used as building blocks to make glucose.

Some amino acids are used to make other products such as ketones, purines and creatine phosphate – a substance well known to athletes, who take creatine supplements to boost muscle strength, especially during weightlifting.

Producing energy from dietary fats

Because the body can only store a small amount of carbohydrate as glycogen for immediate emergency use, glucose is treated as a premium fuel that must be reserved for use by the brain (that's why muscle and fat cells are only 'allowed' to take it up if the hormone insulin is present). So, when possible, your muscle cells use fats as their preferred energy source. Fats are also burned in your liver cells to produce energy – in fact, most of your cells, except brain and mature red blood cells can use fats as an energy source.

Most dietary fats, and your own body-fat stores, are in the form of triglycerides. These have a glycerol backbone to which three fatty acids are attached (to resemble a capital E).

When your glucose levels are low and cells need energy, your pancreas stops making the fat-storage hormone insulin, and instead makes the fat-burning hormone glucagon. As well as telling the liver to start releasing glucose from its glycogen stores, glucagon switches off fat storage and switches on the mobilization of free fatty acids from body fat. It does this indirectly by activating an enzyme known as hormone-sensitive lipase, which breaks down triglycerides into their building blocks of glycerol and free fatty-acid chains. During exercise, and in times of stress, another hormone, adrenaline (epinephrine) made in your adrenal glands also activates hormone-sensitive lipase to release additional fats for energy.

The glycerol released from triglycerides is taken to your liver, where it enters the glycolysis pathway and is broken down to yield a small amount of energy (only 5 per cent of the total energy contained within the triglyceride molecule). The main energy contribution comes from the released free fatty acids. These are transported in your circulation by a blood protein (albumen) and taken to tissues needing energy, such as your skeletal and heart muscle cells. Once escorted inside these cells, the fatty acids are taken into the mitochondria by a transport system called the carnitine shuttle (so called because carnitine is the molecule used to escort the fatty acids inside).

Once within the mitochondria, fatty acids don't feed directly into the citric acid cycle. First, they are processed in a separate series of reactions known as beta-oxidation. During this chain of reactions, molecules of acetyl-coenzyme A are sequentially pinched off the end of the fatty acids. As acetyl-coenzyme A contains only two carbon atoms, a fatty acid such as palmitate, for example, which has a chain of 16 carbon atoms, will yield 8 molecules of acetyl-coenzyme A. Slightly different processes are needed to derive acetyl-coenzyme A from unsaturated fatty acids and from those with an uneven number of carbon atoms, but the end result is the same.

The released acetyl-coenzyme A molecules feed directly into the citric acid cycle (see Diagram 4). Additional NADH and $FADH_2$ are also generated during beta-oxidation. In this way, a molecule of a fatty acid, such as palmitate, yields as much as 104 packets of energy (ATP) compared with the 31 molecules of ATP formed from burning 1 molecule of glucose. As one triglyceride contains three fatty-acid chains plus glycerol, you can see why fat is such an energy-rich storage molecule.

However, there is a down side. Fatty-acid oxidation only delivers this energy at half the rate at which glycogen breakdown supplies energy. So once an athlete uses up his or her glycogen stores during an initial burst of energy, they 'hit the wall' when muscle (and liver) glycogen stores run out. A long-distance runner, for example, is then forced to slow down dramatically once they start burning fat for fuel rather than glucose.

Producing new glucose

The average person has 70 g of carbohydrate stored as glycogen in their liver, and 200 g stored as glycogen in their muscle cells for emergency use. When needed, this glycogen is quickly processed to release glucose. This liver glycogen is enough to see you through the night during your overnight fast so that your brain receives the glucose it needs. During longer periods of not eating, however, you need to raid your protein stores to make energy and glucose instead. Why? Because, as discussed below, you cannot make glucose from your most abundant fuel reserves – the fatty acids within your triglyceride fat stores.

The production of new glucose from non-carbohydrate building blocks such as amino acids (especially alanine), lactate and glycerol (the backbone of triglyceride fats) is known as gluconeogenesis. This process ensures that blood glucose levels remain topped up even when dietary intakes of carbohydrate are low, and your stores of starchy glycogen (in liver and muscle cells) are depleted. Gluconeogenesis mainly occurs in liver cells, but in prolonged starvation it also occurs in the kidney.

The production of glucose is not simply the reverse of the metabolic reactions that broke down glucose to pyruvate (glycolysis), however. Pyruvate must first be converted into oxaloacetate within the mitochondria before following its pathway up to glucose (see Diagram 5). This is important, as it stops you wasting valuable energy in 'futile cycling' where glucose is simultaneously broken down by glycolysis and then remade by gluconeogenesis in the same cell. This mechanism ensures that one or the other pathway takes priority depending on the cells' needs, and is mainly regulated by the amount of glucagon hormone present.

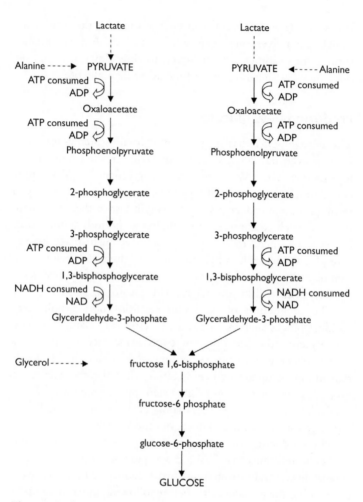

Diagram 5 Chemical steps involved in gluconeogenesis

The conversion of milk and meat proteins to glucose is quite efficient, and your body can make as much as 50 g of glucose from 100 g of these proteins. The liver can also make approximately

10 g of glucose from the glycerol present within 100 g of triglyceride fat. Unfortunately, as mentioned above, it cannot make any net glucose gains from most fatty acids. This is because every time a two-carbon acetyl-coenzyme A splits off from a fatty acid and feeds into the citric acid cycle, two molecules of carbon dioxide are generated as it works its way round the cycle. As a result, there are no spare carbon atoms remaining to act as building blocks for new glucose.

CAN WE OR CAN'T WE?

Some researchers have challenged whether the standard statement that mammals cannot make glucose from fatty acids is really true. Plants and nematodes (roundworms) have enzymes that can convert fatty acids to dicarboxylic acids via a metabolic pathway called the glyoxylate cycle, so they can be used for gluconeogenesis. Some of the enzymes involved have been found in animal tissues, and genes coding for them have also been found in non-placental mammals such as the platypus and the opossum. It's also known that fatty acids with an odd number of carbon atoms, and branched chain fatty acids, can be metabolized to yield succinyl-coenzyme A, which can act as a building block for glucose, but this is not thought to occur in significant amounts.

Energy storage: making glycogen from glucose and vice versa

More often than not, your diet provides excess glucose. When you eat large amounts of carbohydrate in excess of your immediate requirements, it is converted in the liver to the starchy storage molecule glycogen. This process, glycogenesis, is triggered by the presence of the hormone insulin, which is released after a carbohydrate-rich meal.

Glycogen is a complex polymer formed from glucose molecules that are chained together. Branching occurs every ten or so glucose units along the chains, and the whole is wrapped up by a protein, glycogenin, to form a spherical 'blob' inside muscle and liver cells. Glucose is easily snipped off the end of the numerous branches whenever it is needed.

Energy storage: making fat from glucose

As little carbohydrate can be stored as glycogen, excess glucose is converted into fatty acids for storage. This process occurs mainly in the liver cells (hepatocytes) and fat cells (adipocytes). Following pregnancy, it also occurs in breast cells during lactation.

During times of excess, plenty of glucose enters the glycolysis pathway within liver and fat cells. Each molecule of glucose produces two molecules of pyruvate, which enter the cell's mito-chondria and are converted to acetyl-coenzyme A as usual. Acetyl-coenzyme A feeds into the first part of the citric acid cycle by combining with oxaloacetate to make citrate. This is the stage at which the cell has to decide whether to continue pro-cessing it through the citric acid cycle as usual, to produce energy, or whether to divert it for a rainy day and store it as fat. This decision is an easy one for the cell to make. When carbohydrate is plentiful, the mitochondria are already working at full capacity to produce energy and citrate levels build up, forming a bottle-neck in the metabolic pathway. To stop everything clogging up, a control mechanism quickly removes the excess citrate back out of the mitochondria into the main part of the fat cell again. Here, something amazing happens. Increased citrate levels cause the enzymes that promote fatty-acid synthesis to join together, with the vitamin biotin, to form filaments. These filaments act just like factory conveyor belts, converting citrate back into ace-tyl-coenzyme A and joining them together to form fatty-acid chains of various lengths. It has been calculated that a single liver cell can develop as many as 50,000 of these fatty-acid producing filaments at any one time, if needed.

Once formed, the fatty–acid chains are further processed into triglycerides (made up of glycerol plus three fatty acids). In adipose (fat) cells they are stored as a large droplet of fat in the centre of the cell and you gain weight – sometimes at an alarming rate! Fatty acids formed inside liver cells are not usually kept in the liver. They are packaged with protein, to make them soluble, and sent out into the circulation as particles called very low–density lipoprotein (VLDL). Some triglycerides are also obtained from the diet, and are absorbed from the gut (chylomicrons) for transport to fat cells if they are not needed immediately as a fuel. High levels of circulating VLDL and triglycerides can occur on a high-carbohydrate diet and are associated with an increased risk of hardening and furring–up of the arteries, coronary heart disease and stroke.

Although dietary fats are traditionally blamed for raising blood fat levels, it is mainly a high–carbohydrate diet that causes blood triglycerides to rise (in the process described above) in an undesirable way.

FATTY LIVER

If liver cells are hard-pushed from processing lots of carbohydrates, or alcohol, they start to accumulate fat and the liver undergoes fatty change. This is identical to the process involved in the production of pâté de foie gras from force-fed geese and ducks in Perigord, France. Non-alcoholic fatty liver disease (NAFLD) is becoming an increasingly recognized health problem. Some estimates suggest that it affects as many as one in five people, although many cases are mild and remain undiagnosed. It is most common in people who are obese, have Type 2 diabetes or raised triglyceride levels. In some cases, it can progress to cause liver inflammation and scarring.

4
Essential micronutrients: vitamins

Vitamins play a fundamental role in keeping your body's metabolic reactions running smoothly and efficiently. When one or more of these micronutrients are lacking, metabolic reactions may slow down or even fail, so your cells cannot function properly. Despite their importance, most of these micronutrients cannot be made in the body and so must come from your diet. The few that can be made (niacin, vitamin D) are rarely produced in sufficient amounts to meet your needs, and are also classed as 'essential'.

Although vitamins are necessary for health, you only need to obtain tiny amounts from your food. The quantities needed are measured in milligrams (mg) or micrograms (mcg).

VITAMIN UNITS

1 milligram = one thousandth of a gram ($1/1,000$ or 10^{-3} grams)
1 microgram = one millionth of a gram ($1/1,000,000$ or 10^{-6} grams)
1 milligram therefore = 1,000 micrograms.

How do you know how much you need?

Everyone has different, individual needs for each vitamin and mineral, depending on their age, weight, level of activity and the metabolic pathways and enzyme systems they have inherited. Some people need more vitamins and minerals, while some need fewer.

The requirement for each nutrient is therefore calculated according to the best available assessment of average needs. These are calculated using volunteers who undergo a variety of laboratory tests to determine how much of a particular nutrient is needed to maintain a certain blood level or tissue concentration, or how much can prevent signs of deficiency disease.

Different countries take a different approach to setting their recommended daily amounts. One way, used in the UK, is to take the estimated average requirement (EAR) for a particular nutrient and perform some clever number-crunching. First, the statisticians assume that the different needs of everyone in the population form what is known as a normal distribution, with a bell-shaped curve spread on either side of the average. From this distribution, statisticians then work out the standard deviation – a measure of how widely the needs of each individual in the studied population is spread away from the average. A range is then created by taking a value that is two standard deviations on either side of the EAR. This produces a range of intakes that, statistically, encompasses the needs of 95 per cent of the population.

The bottom end of the range (i.e. two standard deviations below the estimated average requirement) is set as the lower-reference nutrient intake (LRNI). Statistically, 2.5 per cent of the studied population will have a low need that is met by this intake, but for 97.5 per cent of the population, this level of intake is inadequate.

The upper level of the range (i.e. two standard deviations above the estimated average intake) is set as the reference nutrient intake (RNI). Statistically, 2.5 per cent of the studied population will have a higher need that is not met by this intake, but for 97.5 per cent of the population, this level of intake is sufficient. This level is therefore set as the reference nutrient intake or recommended daily amount.

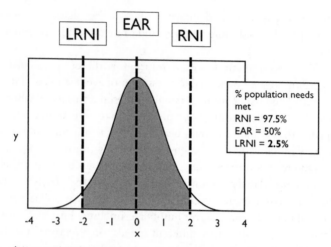

Axis y = number of people Axis x = standard deviations away from the average (mean)

Diagram 6 The normal distribution for nutrient needs. The bell-shaped curve used to determine statistically how much of each nutrient meets the needs of 95 per cent of the population

You may ask why the reference nutrient intake (RNI) is knowingly set so that it will not meet the needs of 2.5 per cent of the population. A good question! Essentially it's because some nutrients may cause toxicity problems for some people – especially those whose needs fall below the LRNI.

A note about deficiencies

In an ideal world, you would get all the vitamins, minerals and essential fatty acids you need from your food. However, we live in the real world where the average adult fails to eat the minimum recommendation of five portions a day of fruit and vegetables, and seven out of ten adults eat no oily fish at all. Even when we do eat reasonable amounts of healthy foods, their nutritional content is often reduced compared with just a generation ago due to being harvested when unripe, then flown to another country and ripened away from its nutrient-absorbing roots.

As a result of poor food choices (cheap processed foods, take-aways) as well as cutting back to lose weight, a surprising number of people are lacking in important vitamins and minerals. This is not always obvious from national assessments of average food intakes because an average is only an average – some will obtain more, while a significant number are getting less. For example,

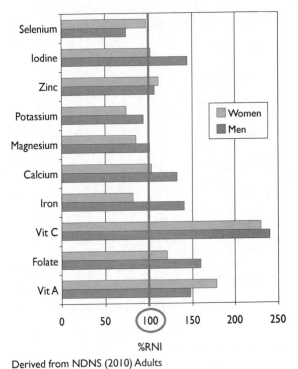

%RNI

Derived from NDNS (2010) Adults

Diagram 7 Average UK intakes of important vitamins and minerals

the most recent National Diet and Nutrition Survey in the UK (2010) suggests that most people are meeting the reference nutrient intake (RNI), or are close to it.

Happy days? Sadly not. These averages hide the fact that a substantial number of adults have intakes that are less than the lower-reference nutrient intake (LRNI). Although 2.5 per cent of people do need intakes that are less than the LRNI, sadly it is usually people with higher needs (especially the elderly) who obtain these lower amounts.

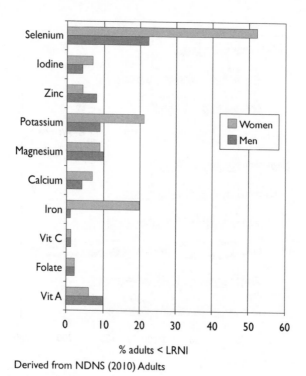

% adults < LRNI

Derived from NDNS (2010) Adults

Diagram 8 Percentage of adults with micronutrient intakes below the LRNI

Many doctors and dieticians claim that micronutrient deficiencies are rare in the developed world. Unfortunately, this is not the case, as the National Diet and Nutrition Survey for 2010 showed. It found that nine out of ten women and eight out of ten children do not obtain recommended amounts of iron; that more than a third of women do not get enough vitamin A, calcium, magnesium, zinc, copper or iodine; that half of men have low intakes of vitamin A and that more than 40 per cent do not obtain enough zinc or magnesium; that 97 per cent of older people do not obtain adequate intakes of nutrients that are vital for good health; that one in four adults have blood levels of vitamin D that are too low for normal bone health. In fact, one in five children in a Southampton study (32 per cent) had vitamin D insufficiency and 8 per cent had overt vitamin D deficiency with bone signs associated with rickets.

In addition to rickets, scurvy, a disease caused by lack of vitamin C, is also making a comeback. In 2004 to 2005, 61 children were admitted to hospital with scurvy in England alone. By 2007 to 2008, this had risen to 94 – a 50 per cent increase.

Another example of micronutrient deficiency involves the mineral selenium. Intakes in Britain almost halved from 60 mcg in 1974 to just 34 mcg per day in 1994 as a result of using European flour for bread-making in place of selenium-rich flour from the United States. Although the full effects of this lack are not yet visible, it is known from other parts of the world with low intakes, such as areas of China, that lack of selenium lowers considerably immunity against viral diseases (e.g. influenza) as well as increasing the risk of Alzheimer's disease, heart muscle weakness and many cancers. In fact, a scientific review of over 150 clinical trials published in the *Journal of the American Medical Association* found that lack of many vitamins is a risk factor for heart disease, stroke, cancer, birth defects, osteoporosis, bone fractures and other major chronic health problems. In an accompanying paper, the authors actually state that: 'Pending strong evidence of effectiveness from randomized trials, it appears prudent for all adults to take vitamin supplements for chronic disease prevention.'

So although severe deficiency diseases such as scurvy are rare, this does illustrate why attention to nutrition is important to help reduce the niggling symptoms (tiredness, dry skin, reduced immunity) that can accompany a minor lack of key micronutrients. Take note of national guidelines, aim to eat your five portions a day of fruit and veg, eat more fish and wholegrains and select locally grown produce that is fresh from the field. If you know your diet is not as good as it could be, a vitamin and mineral supplement is a useful nutritional safety net. You may be surprised to know that, having analysed over a hundred food diaries, I've yet to find someone who gets all the vitamins, minerals and essential fatty acids they need from their food – despite dieticians advising patients that this is possible! In an ideal world, maybe it is. In the real world, it doesn't seem to be the case.

What are vitamins?

Vitamins are molecules that are vital for life. They act as essential intermediaries, or catalysts, to support the enzymes involved in all metabolic reactions in the body. If your intake of any vitamin is low, metabolic deficiencies will eventually result. How quickly these develop depends on the state of your body's stores. You store very little folic acid, for example, so deficiency symptoms may occur within weeks. On the other hand, vitamin B12 is stored in your liver, and it can take years for dietary deficiency to be detected. In general, the fat-soluble vitamins (A, D, E and K) are more readily stored than those that are water-soluble and are easily lost in the urine (vitamin C and most B-group vitamins apart from B12).

The EU Recommended Daily Amount (EU RDA), which is also believed to supply the needs of most (up to 97 per cent) of the adult population are shown in Table 9, together with average

Table 9 Recommended vitamin intakes and upper safe levels for adults aged 18+

Nutrient	EU RDA	Average dietary intakes from food	EVM upper safe level for long-term use from supplements
Vitamins			
Vitamin A (retinol equivalents) (betacarotene)	800 mcg	520 mcg	1,500 mcg[1] 7 mg
Vitamin B1 (thiamin)	1.1 mg	1.5 mg	100 mg
Vitamin B2 (riboflavin)	1.4 mg	1.8 mg	40 mg
Vitamin B3 (niacin)	16 mg	34 mg	500 mg
Vitamin B5 (pantothenic acid)	6 mg	5.4 mg	200 mg
Vitamin B6 (pyridoxine)	1.4 mg	2 mg	10 mg
Vitamin B12 (cobalamin)	2.5 mcg	6.2 mcg	2,000 mcg
Folic acid (folate)	200 mcg[2]	260 mg	1,000 mcg
Biotin	50 mcg	33 mcg	900 mcg
Vitamin C (ascorbic acid)	80 mg	64 mg	1,000 mg
Vitamin D (cholecalciferol)	5 mcg[3]	3 mcg	25 mcg
Vitamin E (tocopherol)	12 mg	8.5 mg	540 mg
Vitamin K	75 mcg	68 mcg	1,000 mcg

[1] This upper safe level refers to total intakes from both diet and supplements

[2] 400 mcg folic acid for women who could become pregnant

[3] For adults confined indoors (no sunlight exposure) and those aged 65 and over, 10 mcg per day is preferable

UK dietary intakes, and upper safe limits suggested by the UK Expert Group on Vitamins and Minerals (EVM) in 2003. The upper safe limits are the maximum daily amount of each vitamin that is considered safe to take long-term in the form of food supplements. These are in addition to the amounts typically obtained from your food, unless otherwise stated. Different RDA values may be used in non-EU countries, and during pregnancy and breastfeeding.

The following sections look at each of the vitamins in turn, explaining what they do, how much you need and the symptoms that can occur when you get too little from your diet. The average dietary intakes quoted are taken from the *Safe Upper Levels for Vitamins and Minerals* report, 2003, from the UK Expert Group on Vitamins and Minerals.

Vitamin A

Vitamin A is not just one, but a group of fat-soluble substances called retinoids. These include retinol and retinyl esters found in animal-based foods, and the plant-based precursors that you can convert into vitamin A such as the yellow pigment betacarotene.

Retinol was named after its first recognized function in the retina of the eye. Here, it is converted into the pigment rhodopsin (visual purple), which is involved in light detection. Vitamin A also acts as an antioxidant, but one of its most important functions is to enter the nucleus of cells where it binds to retinoid nuclear receptors and regulates which genes are switched on to make proteins. So many genes are controlled by vitamin A that it is essential for normal growth, development, immunity, sexual health and fertility. It helps to maintain healthy skin and moist mucous membranes in the lining of the eyes, nose, mouth, lungs and genital tract. It is also needed for healthy bones, teeth, wound healing and the production of immune cells.

Dietary sources of vitamin A

Normally, around 80 per cent of vitamin A in your diet is absorbed in the small intestines, along with dietary fats. Foods containing preformed vitamin A (retinol) include animal and fish liver; meat; oily fish and cod liver oil; eggs; milk and dairy products; butter and fortified margarine.

Foods containing pro-vitamin A carotenoids such as betacarotene, include yellow-orange fruit and vegetables and dark green leafy vegetables.

Vitamin A is easily destroyed by exposure to light, while betacarotene is destroyed by heat and overcooking. Boiling or frying food sources can reduce vitamin A content by 40 per cent after one hour and by 70 per cent after two hours.

Vitamin A is so important for child development that, in many countries including the UK, health officials recommend that children should ideally take a supplement providing vitamins A (together with C and D) at doses appropriate for their age up until at least the age of five. This may not be necessary where their diet is known to provide sufficient amounts of these micronutrients, for example from using a vitamin-enriched formula milk.

INTERNATIONAL UNITS

Vitamin A levels are sometimes given on labels as an International Unit (IU), which is a measure of biological activity rather than weight. This system was developed to take into account the fact that two or more substances may have vitamin A activity in the body (e.g. retinol, betacarotene), and measuring the presence of just one of these would give a false account of dietary intake.

1 IU of Vitamin A = 0.3 mcg retinol
1 mcg vitamin A = 3.33 IU

As it is fat-soluble, vitamin A is readily stored in your liver. Your blood levels are tightly controlled and do not alter substantially until liver stores are severely depleted.

Deficiency

As vitamin A is needed to make a pigment vital for sight (rhodopsin, or visual purple), one of the first signs of lack of vitamin A is loss of sensitivity to green light. This is followed by difficulty in adapting to dim light (night blindness). More severe retinol deficiency leads to dry, burning, itchy eyes, plus corneal hardening and ulceration – a condition known as xerophthalmia. Lack of vitamin A also increases the risk of cataracts. It is estimated that as many as half a million people worldwide go blind from vitamin A deficiency each year. Other symptoms of vitamin A deficiency include growth retardation, reduced male fertility, impaired hearing, taste and smell, increased susceptibility to infection, scaly skin with raised, pimply hair follicles and flaky scalp, loss of appetite and possibly kidney stones.

Vitamin A deficiency is uncommon in developed countries, except in people with reduced absorption, chronic liver disease and alcohol dependency. Worldwide, it is a public health concern in more than half of all countries, especially those in Africa and Asia where general malnutrition is rife and diets include few animal sources of retinol. Worldwide, an estimated 250 million preschool children have a vitamin A deficiency and, as a result, up to half a million children become blind every year, with one in two dying of severe infections within a year of losing their sight. This makes it a leading cause of preventable blindness and death in children. Where deficiency is present, high-dose vitamin A drops can reduce mortality from infections by a quarter overall, while halving the number of deaths associated with acute measles.

Toxicity

Vitamin A has a narrow therapeutic window and intakes of just double the recommended daily amount can cause health problems. As it is fat-soluble, retinol enters the nervous system and excess can cause headache, irritability, blurred vision, nausea, weakness and fatigue. Other symptoms of retinol poisoning include abdominal pain and loss of appetite. In the long term, excess vitamin A may cause hair loss, reduced bone-mineral density and increased risk of liver cirrhosis.

Vitamin A is vital for normal healthy development in the womb, but high intakes during pregnancy (3,000 mcg per day or more) is associated with an increased risk of birth defects, especially when exposure occurs during the first seven weeks of pregnancy. Pregnant women are therefore advised not to take supplements containing preformed retinol (including cod liver oil) or to eat liver products. High doses may also interfere with the function of vitamin K.

> **DANGER!** Avoid eating polar-bear liver, which contains so much retinol that consuming just 100 g can prove lethal.

Vitamin B1

Vitamin B1, also known as thiamin or thiamine, is a water-soluble vitamin that is readily lost via the kidneys. Most people only have stores sufficient to last one month. A regular dietary supply is therefore essential.

Vitamin B1 plays a central role in metabolism as it is needed for an enzyme (pyruvate dehydrogenase) to process pyruvate during the metabolism of glucose (glycolysis). The more carbohydrate you eat, the more thiamin you need. It is also involved in the synthesis of some amino acids, and the function of pancreatic beta cells (which secrete the hormone insulin). It also has a role during nerve-cell stimulation and may be important for regulating mood.

Dietary sources of vitamin B1

Food sources rich in vitamin B1 include unrefined wholegrains and oats; meat products – especially pork and duck; seafood; fruit, nuts and vegetables; dairy products; eggs; pulses, soybean flour; yeast extract.

Vitamin B1 is readily lost into cooking juices during food processing such as chopping, mincing, liquidizing, canning and preserving. Sulphur dioxide, a common preservative in minced meat, destroys 90 per cent thiamin content within two days, while sulphites used to keep processed potatoes white reduce their thiamin content by over 50 per cent. Flour is therefore fortified with thiamin in some countries to replace losses incurred during production. Both baking and toasting bread loses almost a third of its vitamin B1 content, while using baking powder increases losses to 50 per cent.

Boiling reduces the B1 content of foods by half as it leaches into water. It is also destroyed by high temperatures; roasting meat at 200 °C lowers its vitamin B1 content by 20 per cent, while freezing meats reduces their B1 content by up to 50 per cent.

Deficiency

When B1 is lacking, pyruvate accumulates and is converted to lactic acid via anaerobic glycolysis as discussed in Chapter 3. As a result nerve, skeletal and heart muscle cells do not obtain all the energy they need, and their function is reduced.

Thiamin deficiency can develop rapidly, and is common in people with a high alcohol intake (which increases thiamin need) and in parts of the world where the main dietary staple is polished rather than brown rice. Lack of thiamin causes a disease known as *beriberi*, meaning 'extreme weakness', which affects the cardiovascular and nervous systems. Dry beriberi produces heaviness, weakness, numbness and pins and needles in the legs, while wet beriberi causes severe fluid retention. Severe deficiency is associated with a form of dementia, called Wernicke-Korsakoff syndrome, which leads to confusion, unstable gait and even coma if left untreated.

As vitamin B1 is water-soluble, and readily excreted in the urine, toxicity is not an issue.

Vitamin B2

Vitamin B2, or riboflavin, is a water-soluble vitamin that cannot be stored in the body, so a regular dietary intake is essential. B2 plays a crucial role in the production of energy and the metabolism of proteins, fats and carbohydrate during the citric acid cycle. It acts as a building block for the production of flavin adenine dinucleotide (FAD), which carries hydrogen and electrons to the respiratory chain to produce energy (see Chapter 3).

Vitamin B2 plays a key role in growth and the production of glycogen, red blood cells and steroid hormones. It helps insulin-secreting cells in the pancreas to detect the presence of glucose, and is also involved in immunity and the production of antibodies. Other roles include helping to maintain the integrity of your hair, skin, mucous membranes and nails.

Dietary sources of vitamin B2

As it is essential for cell function, vitamin B2 is found in all animal and cell-based foods, especially: yeast extract; liver; lean meats; wholegrain cereals; dairy products; eggs; green leafy vegetables and pulses.

Vitamin B2 is readily lost from vegetables into cooking water, colouring it yellow. Pasteurization of milk loses 20 per cent of its B2 content, which is further reduced by 90 per cent after two hours of sun exposure – buy milk in cartons rather than bottles. Boiling milk also reduces its vitamin B2 content by up to 25 per cent. In addition, freezing meat reduces B2 content by up to 50 per cent.

Deficiency

Severe lack of vitamin B2 (ariboflavinosis) is rare in Western countries, but is occasionally seen in vulnerable groups such as the elderly and those with anorexia or alcohol dependency. Symptoms include a scaly, eczema-like skin rash (seborrhoeic dermatitis), especially on the face and nose, sensitivity to bright light, itching, dizziness, insomnia, slow learning, weakness, sore and swollen throat and tongue, cracking and sores at the corners of the mouth (angular cheilosis), bloodshot corneas and anaemia.

Vitamin B2 is relatively non-toxic as excess is readily excreted in the urine.

Vitamin B3

Vitamin B3, or niacin, occurs in two main forms, both of which are water-soluble: nicotinic acid and nicotinamide, which is the active form. Small amounts of B3 can be made in the body from the essential amino acid tryptophan (60 mg tryptophan produces 1 mg niacin). Because of this, the vitamin B3 content of foods and supplements is sometimes given as 'niacin equivalents', which are equal to the amount of nicotinamide and nicotinic acid they contain plus one-sixtieth of their tryptophan content.

B3 plays a crucial role in the production of energy and the metabolism of proteins, fats and carbohydrates during the citric acid cycle. It acts as a building block for the production of nicotinamide adenine dinucleotide (NAD) and nicotinamide adenine dinucelotide phosphate (NADP). These act as coenzymes, which activate over 200 dehydrogenase enzymes involved in energy production and electron transport in cells as discussed in Chapter 3. NADP is also involved in the synthesis of fatty acids, steroid hormones and a sugar, called ribose, which forms part of your genetic material (DNA). People who are physically active therefore need more niacin than sedentary people.

Vitamin B3 regulates the production of triglycerides and 'good' HDL-cholesterol in your liver. It also combines with the mineral chromium to form a substance that is commonly known as Glucose Tolerance Factor (GTF), as it increases insulin binding and glucose uptake into cells. As a B vitamin, its other important roles include helping to maintain healthy skin and nerve function.

Dietary sources of vitamin B3

Dietary sources of B3 include: wholegrains; meat and poultry; oily fish; dairy products; nuts; dried fruit and yeast extract.

Eggs and cheese are among the richest dietary sources of tryptophan.

Deficiency

Lack of vitamin B3 produces a rare deficiency disease known as pellagra, meaning raw skin, which classically produces symptoms of dermatitis (in sun-exposed areas of the body), diarrhoea and dementia plus fatigue, sleeplessness, depression, memory loss and visual impairment. This is mainly seen in parts of Africa where the diet contains large quantities of maize, whose niacin is in a non-usable form of niacytin. In Central America, however, maize for cooking tortillas is soaked overnight in calcium hydroxide, which releases the niacin content.

Toxicity

High doses of B3, especially in the form of nicotinic acid, can produce facial flushing. Very high intakes can cause thickening and darkening of skin (acanthosis nigricans), palpitations, peptic ulceration, gout and hepatitis.

Vitamin B5

Vitamin B5, or pantothenic acid, is a water-soluble vitamin that is a vital component of coenzyme A, which is involved in the citric acid cycle as acetyl-coenzyme A and succinyl-coenzyme A. Vitamin B5 is therefore vital for many energy-producing reactions in the body involving carbohydrates, fats and proteins. It is needed to synthesize glucose, fatty acids and adrenal hormones. It also stimulates cell growth in healing tissues, increasing the number and speed of cells moving into wounds and promoting stronger scar-tissue formation.

Dietary sources of vitamin B5

Rich sources include: poultry, meat, offal; wholegrains; eggs, especially fish roes; vegetables, especially broccoli, potatoes and tomatoes; pulses and yeast extract.

Despite its wide distribution, vitamin B5 is easily destroyed by food processing. Cooking destroys up to 50 per cent of B5 present in meats, and an additional 30 per cent is lost into cooking juices. Up to 75 per cent of B5 in vegetables is lost during processing and freezing.

Deficiency

Vitamin B5 deficiency is very rare, but can include irritability, restlessness, fatigue, apathy, malaise, sleep disturbance, nausea, vomiting, abdominal cramps and symptoms of the nervous system such as numbness, tingling sensations, muscle cramps, staggering gait and burning sensations in the feet. Low blood-glucose levels and an increased sensitivity to insulin have also been recorded.

Vitamin B6

Vitamin B6 consists of three water-soluble compounds: pyridox-ine, pyridoxal and pyridoxamine that are converted into the most active form, pyridoxine, within the liver. Small amounts are stored in the liver, muscle tissue and brain.

Pyridoxine is an essential cofactor for the action of over 60 enzymes involved in the synthesis of genetic material, amino acids, proteins and the metabolism of carbohydrates and essential fatty acids. It is especially needed by rapidly dividing cells such as those found in the gut, skin, hair follicles and marrow. It is involved in the production of antibodies, hydrochloric acid in the stomach, the synthesis of brain neurotransmitters and in the sodium–potassium balance. It can affect mental processing and mood, and modify the action of sex hormones. It is also neces-sary for breaking down homocysteine – an amino acid that can damage blood-vessel walls to hasten the hardening and furring-up of the arteries (atherosclerosis). Vitamin B6 requires the pres-ence of vitamin B2, zinc and magnesium as cofactors to fulfil all its physiological functions.

Dietary sources of vitamin B6

Rich sources of vitamin B6 include: meat, especially liver; oily fish; egg yolk; wholegrain cereals, especially brown rice; soy products; nuts, especially peanuts and walnuts; green, leafy vege-tables and yeast extract.

Up to 70 per cent of vitamin B6 in meat is lost during processing and cooking. Sterilization reduces pyridoxine in milk by 20 per cent, canning lowers vegetable pyridoxine by 20 per cent and a further 40 per cent is lost into water when frozen vegetables are thawed and cooked.

Deficiency

Lack of vitamin B6 is uncommon but has been associated with depression, irritability, a greasy rash on the forehead and around the nose plus cracking of the lips and tongue. Deficiency has also been linked with carpal tunnel syndrome, and symptoms similar to those occurring in premenstrual syndrome (PMS) such as anxiety, irritability, mild depression, bloating and tender breasts. Although this is controversial, supplements are sometimes recommended for women experiencing debilitating PMS symptoms.

Toxicity

High doses of vitamin B6 may cause headache, acne, skin reactions, nausea, abdominal pain, loss of appetite and can cause abnormal results in liver-function tests. There have been some suggestions that prolonged high doses, of above 10 mg daily, may cause reversible nerve symptoms such as pins and needles, but this is controversial. The risks associated with taking vitamin B6 at doses between 10 mg and 200 mg long term are unclear, but are probably low.

Vitamin B12

Vitamin B12, also known as cobalamin, is a micronutrient that contains cobalt – the only known requirement for this metal in human physiology. Although water-soluble, you can store enough in your liver to last several years.

Vitamin B12 acts as a cofactor for enzymes involved in fatty-acid and amino-acid metabolism and the processing of homocysteine – a potentially harmful amino acid linked with atherosclerosis. It is essential when genetic material (DNA) is synthesized during cell division, and if in short supply, newly formed cells are larger than usual. When this affects red blood cells, pernicious anaemia results. When it occurs during pregnancy, developmental abnormalities such as spina bifida are possible. Pregnant women have recently been advised to take vitamin B12 supplements together with their folic acid. Other key roles for vitamin B12 include helping to maintain normal nerve function, immunity and healing.

Dietary sources of vitamin B12

B12 is only found in consistent amounts in animal-based foods such as: liver and kidney; meat and poultry; oily fish, especially sardines; eggs and dairy products.

Vegetarian sources include blue-green algae, extracts from bacterial cultures and synthetic B12 in fortified breakfast cereals. Around 20 per cent of the B12 in food leaches out into juices during cooking.

Deficiency

Vitamin B12 is absorbed in the lower part of the small intestine, but only if a carrier protein, gastric intrinsic factor, is present (which is made by cells in the stomach lining). Vitamin B12 deficiency becomes increasingly common with age due to loss of the cells that produce intrinsic factor, and/or reduced absorption in the small intestine because of bowel disease. People with autoimmune conditions such as Type 1 diabetes and thyroid disease are especially likely to develop B12 deficiency, due to autoimmune loss of intrinsic-factor function. B12 absorption also depends on the presence of calcium.

Lack of vitamin B12 causes the production of cells that are larger than they should be. In the case of red blood cells, this leads to a particular form of anaemia known as pernicious anaemia. As this develops slowly and gradually, the symptoms, including paleness (often with a lemon tinge to the skin), tiredness, weakness and shortness of breath, are often not recognized until the anaemia is advanced.

Vitamin B12 is also needed for healthy nerve function and if not recognized and treated, deficiency can damage nerves in the spinal cord, leading to a rare condition known as subacute combined degeneration of the spinal cord. Other symptoms that may be caused by a vitamin B12 deficiency include a smooth, sore tongue, tiredness, exhaustion, menstrual disorders, numbness, tingling, trembling, clumsiness, difficulty walking (especially in the dark when you can't see where you are going), poor memory, lack of concentration, confusion and depression.

Because the symptoms are so variable, vitamin B12 deficiency should be considered in all spinal-cord, nerve and psychiatric disorders. Many people who are lacking in B12 do not develop obvious symptoms for several years, however, and they tend to creep up on you slowly in an insidious way – hence the name of the vitamin B12 deficiency disease, 'pernicious' anaemia. Although vitamin B12 treatment for pernicious anaemia traditionally involves intramuscular injections, it can be given sublingually (under the tongue) in high doses as absorption through oral mucus membranes overcomes the lack of intestinal intrinsic factor.

Itchy rash and diarrhoea have been reported at high doses.

Biotin

Biotin is a water-soluble B-group vitamin. It is an essential cofactor for acetyl-coenzyme A and related compounds, and for carboxylase enzymes involved in the synthesis and metabolism of fatty acids, glucose and amino acids. Biotin may also play a role in gene expression, stimulate insulin secretion from pancreatic beta cells and promote the activity of glucose receptors (Glut-4) which transport glucose into muscle and fat cells when insulin is present. Biotin is also important for healthy hair, skin, nails and sweat glands.

Dietary sources of biotin

These include liver; meat; oily fish; egg yolk and yeast extract. Biotin is also produced by probiotic bacteria in yogurt and in your own bowel, from which you can absorb useful amounts.

Deficiency

As biotin is widely distributed in food, and is also made by bacteria in the gut, from which it can be absorbed, dietary deficiency is rare. It can occur in those taking long-term antibiotics (e.g. for acne), although probiotic supplements will help to overcome this effect. Biotin deficiency can also occur in bodybuilders who eat large amounts of raw egg white over a long period. Raw (but not cooked) egg white contains the protein avidin, that binds to biotin and prevents its absorption.

Lack of biotin can cause dry, scaly, flaky skin, a rash around the nose and mouth, brittle hair and nails, patchy hair loss, tiredness and loss of appetite. Around one in 120 people have an inherited, inborn error of biotin metabolism. This is believed to affect their immunity against yeast infections and may be linked with recurrent candida infections.

Biotin is non-toxic as any excess is excreted in the urine.

Folate

Folates are a group of water-soluble compounds that are sometimes referred to as vitamin B9. Their name is derived from the Latin word *folium* meaning 'leaf', as this is where the first folate was identified. Folates containing more than one glutamate are absorbed and used less efficiently in the body than the synthetic monoglutamate form known as folic acid.

Folic acid is involved in the synthesis and metabolism of proteins, sugar and nucleic acids. Together with vitamin B12, it is especially important for cells that are dividing rapidly. When folic acid is in short supply, dividing cells become unusually large and, when red blood cells are affected, anaemia results.

Folic acid is essential during the first few weeks of a baby's development in the womb. Deficiency can trigger a type of developmental abnormality known as a neural tube defect (for example, spina bifida), which arises between the twenty-fourth and twenty-eighth day after conception.

Folate is also needed to process an amino acid, homocysteine, raised levels of which are associated with atherosclerosis. Two of the three enzymes that control homocysteine levels depend on folate for their activity.

Dietary sources of folate

Folate-rich food sources include green leafy vegetables, e.g. spinach, broccoli, Brussels sprouts, parsley; wholegrains; beans and soy products; liver and kidney; citrus fruit; nuts; dairy products; eggs and yeast extract.

Foods originally rich in folate typically retain less than a third of their folate content after processing and cooking. Folate is destroyed by prolonged contact with light and air but can be protected by antioxidant vitamin C. Up to 90 per cent of folate content of grain is lost during milling, 10 per cent of folate in vegetables is lost by steaming, 20 per cent by pressure-cooking and up to 50 per cent by boiling.

Women planning for a baby are advised to take daily supplements containing 400 mcg folic acid from before the time of conception and during at least the first 12 weeks of pregnancy. Considerably higher doses of 4 mg per day are advised for women with a personal or family history of conceiving a child with a neural tube defect. Folic acid supplements are generally considered safe, but long-term use of high doses can mask vitamin B12 deficiency, as it prevents the occurrence of red blood cell changes that allow a lack of vitamin B12 to be detected. Therefore, the upper safe level for long-term use from supplements is suggested as 1,000 mcg (1 mg) daily, except for certain women, during pregnancy.

Deficiency

The body stores very little folic acid, and dietary lack rapidly causes deficiency – it is cited as the most widespread vitamin deficiency in developed countries. Lack of folic acid results in reduced DNA synthesis and impaired cell division, which is usually detected due to the resulting macrocytic (large-cell) anaemia. Symptoms of folic acid deficiency include a red, sore tongue, tiredness, exhaustion, cracking at the corners of the mouth and weakness. Vitamin B12 deficiency can be masked by taking folate supplements, so these two supplements are usually given together.

Vitamin C

Vitamin C, or ascorbic acid, is a water-soluble vitamin that cannot be stored in the body in appreciable amounts. Its chemical structure is related to glucose, but unlike most animals, which can synthesize vitamin C from glucose and galactose, humans and other primates lack the enzyme (L-gulonolactone oxidase) needed to make their own supplies.

MEMBERS OF THE EXCLUSIVE VITAMIN-C-FREE CLUB

The only animals unable to synthesize vitamin C are:

- man and other primates
- guinea pigs
- Indian fruit bat
- red-vented bulbul (an Asian songbird)
- rainbow trout
- Coho salmon
- a single strain of Japanese laboratory rat

The goat, for example, which weighs around the same as a man, produces between 2 g and 13 g of vitamin C per day depending on its levels of stress and illness.

Vitamin C is an important antioxidant in all body tissues, especially the eye lens. It also regenerates other antioxidants, such as vitamin E, which initially become free radicals themselves after performing their antioxidant function. The highest concentrations are found in the adrenal glands, pituitary gland and the retina of the eyes. Vitamin C acts as an essential cofactor for at least 300 metabolic reactions which are promoted when large quantities of vitamin C are available. It is essential for conversion of the amino acid proline to hydroxyproline during collagen synthesis. It is also involved in the metabolism of stress hormones and the regulation of immune reactions.

The presence of vitamin C increases the absorption of iron in the gut by converting ferric iron (Fe^{3+}) to ferrous iron (Fe^{2+}) – for more details of this process, see the next chapter on minerals.

Dietary sources of vitamin C

Vitamin C is mainly found in fruit and vegetables such as black-currants, berries, guava, kiwi fruit, citrus fruit, mango, capsicum peppers, green leafy vegetables and potatoes. Animal sources include kidney and liver.

Vitamin C is one of the most unstable vitamins, and up to two-thirds is lost through processing, prolonged cooking and storage. Fruit juices rapidly lose their vitamin C content when exposed to air, even if chilled – virtually all is lost within 14 days. Cooking soft fruits removes two-thirds of their vitamin C content; when boiled, vegetables lose up to 50 per cent of vitamin C into the cooking water and during storage; and root vegetables lose around 10 per cent of vitamin C content per month. Some vegetables, such as asparagus, lose 90 per cent of their vitamin C content after just one week.

The EU RDA for vitamin C was recently increased from 60 mg to 80 mg, based on new understandings of average metabolic needs. In the US, the recommended intake is higher for adult males (90 mg) but slightly lower for women (75 mg). Smokers are advised to obtain 35 mg per day more, due to the oxidative damage caused by toxins in cigarette smoke, which lower blood levels of vitamin C.

Deficiency

The absorption and metabolism of vitamin C varies depending on the amount consumed. At intakes of up to 200 mg as a single dose, absorption of vitamin C is almost complete through an active transport process. At single doses of over 500 mg, it is also absorbed through a process of diffusion, which is less efficient so that only around half of a 1.5 g dose is absorbed and only 16 per cent of a massive 12 g dose.

Mild deficiency of vitamin C is relatively common, and is associated with non-specific symptoms (sometimes known as pre-scurvy syndrome) such as frequent colds and other infections, lack of energy, weakness and muscle and joint pain.

More severe lack of vitamin C leads to a deficiency disease known as scurvy. A minimum daily intake of 10 mg vitamin C is needed to prevent this, although 20 mg per day is needed for normal wound healing. In scurvy, reduced conversion of the amino acid proline to hydroxyproline (an important component of collagen) results in poor wound healing; dry, rough, scaly skin; broken thread veins in skin around hair follicles; easy bruising; scalp dryness; misshapen, tangled, corkscrew, brittle hair; hair loss; dry, fissured lips; inflamed, spongy, bleeding gums and loose teeth; bleeding skin, eyes and nose and muscle weakness.

Toxicity

The safety of vitamin C supplementation has been researched and established over a long period of time. Some vitamin C is metabolized to oxalic acid, but claims that large doses could trigger oxalate kidney stones have proved unfounded. However, those known to be recurrent stone-formers who have a defect in ascorbic acid or oxalate metabolism and people with renal failure should restrict daily vitamin C intakes to approximately 100 mg.

Large doses may trigger indigestion or diarrhoea. This is largely due to the acidity of vitamin C rather than a specific sign of toxicity, and some people are more sensitive to the acidity of vitamin C than others.

WARNINGS

Individuals with the iron-storage disease haemochromatosis should not take vitamin C supplements except under medical advice.

> Suddenly stopping high-dose supplements can cause temporary symptoms of vitamin C deficiency (rebound scurvy), when enzymes activated by high levels of vitamin C are suddenly deprived of the extra vitamin C they need to work properly.

Vitamin D

Vitamin D, or calciferol, is the collective term for five different fat-soluble vitamins, of which the most important are vitamin D2 (ergocalciferol, derived from plant foods), and vitamin D3 (cholecalciferol, derived from animal foods). Dietary vitamin D3 is significantly more effective in maintaining blood vitamin D levels than vitamin D2.

MAKING IT ON YOUR OWN

Vitamin D3 can be synthesized photochemically in your skin from a reaction between 7-dehydrocholesterol and UVB ultraviolet sunlight (290 nm to 315 nm spectrum). This only occurs when the UV index is greater than 3 which, in the UK, is achieved during spring and summer. You cannot produce enough vitamin D to meet your needs during autumn and winter, when your blood levels of vitamin D naturally tend to fall. Used properly, a sunscreen with a sun protection factor of SPF8 reduces vitamin D production in the skin by 95 per cent, while SPF15 reduces vitamin D production by 99 per cent. The development of a tan suggests enough UVB radiation has struck the skin to stimulate production of melanin pigment and some vitamin D, regardless of sunscreen use.

Cholecalciferol is classed as a prohormone, as your liver and kidneys convert it into the hormone calcitriol (1,25-dihydroxycholecalciferol). Calcitriol regulates calcium and phosphate metabolism via the kidneys, small intestines and bone by increasing calcium and phosphorus absorption in the small intestines, regulating calcium reabsorption in the kidneys as well as the secretion of parathyroid hormone, which releases calcium from bones.

In addition, vitamin D regulates the balance between production and breakdown of bone and joint connective tissues such as collagen and elastin during bone growth and remodelling. It stimulates the production of proteoglycans (cartilage building blocks) within joints and stimulates immune cells that fight infection and target cancer cells.

Recent research also suggests that vitamin D plays a direct role in learning, memory and mood – especially in older people – as well as reducing calcium deposition in arteries to reduce hardening of the arteries (arteriosclerosis).

Dietary sources of vitamin D

Vitamin D is mainly obtained from eating: oily fish (sardine, herring, mackerel, salmon, tuna); fish-liver oils; liver; eggs; fortified milk; fortified margarine and butter.

The EU RDA for vitamin D is 5 mcg. People over the age of 50 usually need at least 10 mcg per day as blood levels fall with increasing age and synthesis in the skin becomes less efficient. The upper safe level for long-term use from supplements is suggested as 25 mcg per day in the UK, although this is generally considered too low. An upper safe level of 50 mcg has been suggested by the US Food and Nutrition Board and the European Commission Scientific Committee on Food, while an upper safe level of 80 mcg per day has been set in Australia and New Zealand.

Vitamin D amounts are sometimes expressed as a measure of activity (International Units, or IU) rather than as a measure of weight (micrograms) as different molecules contribute to vitamin D status in the body. Each 1 mcg of vitamin D is equivalent to 40 IU. The EU RDA of 5 mcg is therefore equivalent to 200 IU per day.

Deficiency

Vitamin D deficiency occurs in those who do not obtain or absorb enough from their diet and do not regularly expose their skin to sunlight – either because they are confined indoors or because they cover their skin with clothing or sunblock. Prolonged vitamin D deficiency in children results in rickets. In adults, vitamin D deficiency results in osteomalacia with softening of bones, skeletal pain, increased risk of fractures and muscle weakness. These changes are due to raised levels of parathyroid hormone, which leaches calcium from bones. Increased calcium in the circulation may become deposited in coronary artery walls and contribute to heart disease. Lack of vitamin D has recently been linked with reduced immunity and an increased risk of bacterial vaginosis in pregnancy, a common bacterial imbalance that increases the risk of miscarriage and premature labour.

Toxicity

Excess vitamin D can cause headache, loss of appetite, nausea, vomiting, diarrhoea or constipation, palpitations and fatigue.

Vitamin E

Vitamin E is the collective term for two groups of fat-soluble compounds: the tocopherols and tocotrienols. These consist of four tocopherols (alpha, beta, gamma and delta) and four tocotrienols (alpha, beta, gamma and delta). Recently, a ninth substance with vitamin E activity, delta-tocomonoenol, was identified in kiwi fruit. Of all of these, the most active form is natural source d-alpha-tocopherol. Synthetic d-alpha tocopherol is less biologically active due to the different molecular symmetries present. Total vitamin E activity is therefore usually expressed as d-alpha-tocopherol equivalents. Alpha-tocopherol is the main source of vitamin E in the European diet, while gamma-tocopherol is the most common form in the American diet.

Vitamin E mainly functions as an antioxidant in the lipid (fatty) parts of the body, maintaining the integrity of cell membranes, nerve sheaths, circulating cholesterol molecules, dietary fats and body fat stores. When it acts as an antioxidant it is itself converted into a free radical and other antioxidants, such as vitamin C, are needed to regenerate antioxidant vitamin E. Like vitamin A, vitamin E may also modify gene expression and transcription to strengthen muscle fibres and boost immunity. Interestingly, selenium and vitamin E appear to have a synergistic effect to increase antibody synthesis.

Dietary sources of vitamin E

These include: wheatgerm, soybean, corn and olive oils; avocado; butter and fortified margarine; wholegrain cereals; nuts and seeds; meat, poultry and dairy products.

Vitamin E is rapidly depleted on exposure to air. Processing cereals and grains, canning vegetables and freezing removes over 80 per cent of their vitamin E content. Heating destroys around 30 per cent of vitamin E content of foods, while frying or roasting destroys virtually all vitamin E present.

Vitamin E activity is sometimes expressed in International Units (IU) rather than milligrams, as nine different chemicals contribute towards vitamin E activity in the body. One IU = 0.67 mg alpha-tocopherol equivalents, or conversely: 1 mg = 1.5 IU. The EU RDA for vitamin E of 12 mg is therefore equivalent to 18 IU. In general, the more polyunsaturated fats you eat, the more vitamin E you need.

Deficiency

Lack of vitamin E affects the integrity of cell membranes, muscle contraction and nerve transmission. As a result, lack of vitamin E has a harmful effect on the nervous system and can produce symptoms such as lack of energy, lethargy, poor concentration, irritability, muscle weakness and poor coordination. In severe, long-term lack (such as that incurred by malabsorption) serious effects such as blindness, dementia and abnormal heart rhythms can occur.

Toxicity

Vitamin E is relatively non-toxic. Very high intakes can cause headache, fatigue, double vision, muscle weakness, abdominal pain and diarrhoea. High doses may also interfere with the function of vitamin K.

Vitamin K

Vitamin K is the collective term for a group of four fat-soluble substances: phylloquinone (K1 made in plants), menaquinone (K2, made by Gram-positive bacteria in your small intestine) plus menadione (K3) and menadiol (K4), which are closely related synthetic substances found to have vitamin K activity (although they are not present in nature).

Vitamin K was named after the German word *koagulation,* as it acts as an essential cofactor for the production of certain blood-clotting proteins in the liver: factors II (prothrombin), VII, IX, X, protein C, protein S and protein Z. It therefore acts as an antidote for the blood-thinning drug warfarin. Vitamin K is also needed for the synthesis of osteocalcin (a calcium-binding protein found in bone), and plays a role in the reabsorption of calcium in the kidneys. It is also thought to play a role in cell signalling, brain metabolism and cardiovascular health.

Dietary sources of vitamin K

Most of your vitamin K requirements are met by probiotic bacteria in your gut, which secrete absorbable vitamin K2. Dietary sources, of which 90 per cent are in the form of vitamin K1, include cauliflower (the richest source); dark green leafy vegetables; safflower, rapeseed, soybean and olive oils; fish-liver oils; yogurt; dairy products; meat and eggs.

Deficiency

As it is secreted by intestinal bacteria, deficiency is rare but can occur as a result of malabsorption or prolonged use of broad-spectrum antibiotics. Symptoms that may be due to lack of vitamin K include prolonged bleeding time, easy bruising, recurrent nosebleeds, heavy periods and diarrhoea. A single dose of vitamin K is offered to all newborn infants to prevent a condition known as haemorrhagic disease of the newborn.

High doses of vitamins A or E may interfere with vitamin K function.

Toxicity

Patients taking warfarin should avoid extreme changes to dietary intake of vitamin K from vegetables such as broccoli or cauliflower, which can affect blood-clotting control. However, as long as you maintain a fairly consistent intake of these foods, and your warfarin tests are stabilized to that intake, you do not need to avoid them altogether.

5

Essential micronutrients: minerals and trace elements

Essential minerals are metallic and non-metallic elements that play a vital role in body metabolism. Those needed in very tiny amounts are usually referred to as trace elements.

Despite the fact that you store over 3 kg of minerals within your skeleton, mineral deficiency is generally more common than vitamin deficiency. Unlike the vitamin content of a particular food, which is usually similar wherever it is harvested, the mineral content of your food depends on the soil in which its ingredients were grown or reared. This is because plant roots absorb vital nutrients from the soil for optimum growth and these, in turn, are eaten by livestock. Selenium, for example, was leached out of the soil throughout much of Europe during the last Ice Age. Exposure to acid rain, which can interact with minerals to form insoluble salts, and food processing can also significantly reduce the mineral content of foods.

Minerals have several different functions in the body. Some act as antioxidants (selenium, manganese, zinc), while others have structural roles (calcium, magnesium, phosphate). Some maintain electrical potentials across cell membranes (sodium, potassium, chloride), and are vital for electrical transmission in muscle and nerve cells and muscle contraction (calcium). Many act as cofactors for important enzymes (copper, iron, magnesium, manganese, molybdenum, selenium, zinc), or are important for hormone function (chromium, iodine). Perhaps the best known, however, is iron, which forms part of the proteins that bind oxygen in red blood cells (haemoglobin) and muscle cells (myoglobin).

As discussed at the beginning of the previous chapter, the EU Recommended Daily Amounts (EU RDA) estimate the intake of minerals and trace elements that are believed to supply the needs of most (97.5 per cent) of the adult population. These are shown in Table 10, together with the upper safe limits suggested by the UK Expert Group on Vitamins and Minerals (EVM) in 2003. To recap, the upper safe limits are the maximum daily amount of each mineral that is considered safe to take long term in the form of food supplements. These are in addition to the amounts typically obtained from your food, unless otherwise stated. Different RDA values are used in non-EU countries, and during pregnancy and breastfeeding.

Table 10 Recommended mineral intakes and upper safe levels for adults aged 18 and over

Mineral for which an EU RDA has been set	EU RDA	Average dietary intakes from food	EVM upper safe level for long-term use from supplements
Minerals			
Calcium	800 mg	830 mg per day from food; up to 600 mg from water	1,500 mg
Chloride	800 mg	up to 6,000 mg	Not suggested
Chromium	40 mcg	100 mcg per day	10 mg[1]

(*Continued*)

Table 10 Cont'd

Mineral for which an EU RDA has been set	EU RDA	Average dietary intakes from food	EVM upper safe level for long-term use from supplements
Copper	1 mg	1.4 mg per day from food, and up to 6 mg per day from water	10 mg[1]
Iodine	150 mcg	250 mcg per day	500 mcg
Iron	14 mg	12 mg per day	17 mg
Magnesium	375 mg	380 mg per day	400 mg
Manganese	2 mg	5 mg	4 mg
Phosphorus	700 mg	1,260 mg per day	250 mg
Potassium	2,000 mg	2,800 mg per day	3,700 mg
Selenium	55 mcg	39 mcg per day	350 mcg
Zinc	10 mg	9.8 mg per day from food, and up to 10 mg per day from water	25 mg

[1] This upper safe level refers to total intakes from both diet and supplements

A word on bioavailability

Vitamins and minerals are absorbed from the small intestine, mainly within the jejunum. Their bioavailability refers to the fraction that is ingested and absorbed to become available for your body to use or store. The proportion of vitamins and minerals in the diet that is absorbed varies from person to person, and can also change over time. The absorption of many minerals in particular (e.g. chromium) is inefficient and highly variable, while for others efficiency can be high. For example, as much as 98 per cent of the selenium present in some food sources is absorbed.

Once ingested, minerals are mainly absorbed into intestinal lining cells (enterocytes) via passive diffusion. Some minerals also enter intestinal cells by following the movement of water (solvent drag) by squeezing between intestinal cells (e.g. magnesium) or by a process called cell drinking (pinocytosis) in which part of the cell encloses and engulfs a small droplet of fluid (e.g. calcium). These processes are unregulated, and you absorb the nutrients whether you need them or not.

Important minerals such as phosphorus, magnesium and zinc are also absorbed by a regulated process called active transport, which boosts uptake when intake is low or demand is high.

The absorption of many minerals depends on acidity (pH), and low levels of stomach acid (achlorhydria), which becomes increasingly common as you get older, can lead to a number of nutritional deficiencies, especially of zinc and of calcium, which also depends on the presence of vitamin D.

The chemical form in which minerals are presented to intestinal lining cells also affects their uptake. Most dietary iron is in the form of inorganic ferrous iron (Fe^{2+}) or ferric iron (Fe^{3+}), for example. Ferrous iron has a relatively inefficient uptake mechanism but when vitamin C (ascorbic acid) is present, it is converted into ferric iron, which is better absorbed due to its higher solubility. In contrast, the iron present in meat (haem iron) is 'body ready', as it is bound to porphyrin which is absorbed via a specific haem receptor, that is two to three times more efficient. Even so, only around 10 to 15 per cent of the iron present in a varied diet is usually absorbed.

Previous intake and body status

Mineral absorption may depend on previous intakes and how much is stored in the body (tissue saturation). Iron, for example, is initially stored within intestinal lining cells bound to a protein called ferritin, which releases it as needed. Once a cell's ferritin is saturated with iron, it does not absorb more iron from food within the gut. Iron can only leave enterocytes and enter the circulation by binding to a blood protein called transferrin. If circulating transferrin saturation is high, iron remains within the enterocytes and is lost when the intestinal cell is shed (which occurs, on average, after a lifespan of three days). As absorption is inversely related to body iron stores, those with iron deficiency absorb more. This mechanism helps to prevent absorption of excess iron, which can be harmful. Similarly, movement of zinc depends on a protein, metallothionein, which 'traps' zinc within intestinal lining cells when body stores are high.

Gut health

Disorders that hasten gut transit time (e.g. diarrhoea from gastro-enteritis, irritable bowel syndrome) will reduce mineral absorption, while a slowed gut transit time (e.g. constipation) may increase absorption due to prolonged contact between minerals and intestinal lining cells.

Gut diseases such as Crohn's disease and ulcerative colitis can also affect absorption – either reducing uptake through active transport mechanisms or increasing passive diffusion by disrupting the integrity of the intestinal lining.

Other dietary components

Mineral absorption is influenced by the presence of other dietary compounds within the intestines. Substances that bind to minerals (chelators) such as bran and phytic acid (found especially in unleavened wheat bread) can hold them within the intestines so that they remain unabsorbed. Phytic acid, for example, has been reported to inhibit the absorption of iron, zinc, calcium and manganese but not of copper. Polyphenols, such as tannic acid found in tea and some vegetables, also chelate iron and other minerals. Similarly, free fatty acids can form insoluble soaps with calcium and magnesium to impair their absorption, while an as yet unidentified component of coffee appears to inhibit iron absorption.

Minerals can interfere with the absorption of each other, too. Iron interferes with zinc absorption, while copper uptake is impaired by the presence of zinc, iron and molybdenum.

As the previous pages have shown, simply measuring the amount of minerals (or vitamins) present in the diet is not always enough when assessing your diet, as there is no guarantee of how much of each micronutrient is absorbed. Blood testing in order to measure the micronutrient status of the body may be needed when nutritional deficiencies are suspected.

Boron

Boron is a non-metallic trace element that is abundant in oceans, rocks and some soils. Its function is not fully understood, but it interacts with several enzymes to stimulate or inhibit their action. As such, it is believed to promote chemical transmission in the brain and to boost the production of active vitamin D and the hormones oestrogen and testosterone.

Dietary sources of boron

Boron is essential for plant health and is present in nuts; fruit, especially apples, grapes, pears, plums, prunes, strawberries and avocado, and green vegetables, especially broccoli. Small amounts are also present in drinking water.

No EU RDA for boron has been set. The World Health Organization suggests intakes of between 1 mg and 13 mg per day are adequate.

Deficiency

Lack of boron is believed to contribute to a rare form of joint deformity known as Kashin-Beck disease that is also linked to selenium deficiency. Some researchers have also suggested that osteoporosis is a boron-deficiency disease, though this is controversial.

Toxicity

Symptoms of toxicity may include headache, muscle pain, nausea, vomiting, red eyes, rash and desquamation (peeling skin).

Calcium

Calcium is an alkaline metal and is the most abundant mineral in your body. Almost all your stores (around 1.2 kg) are in your bones and teeth in the form of calcium phosphate (hydroxyapatite) embedded in a collagen protein framework. The 1 per cent that is outside your skeleton is vital for life, however, as it is involved in energy production, muscle contraction (including your heartbeat), nerve conduction, immune function and blood clotting.

Absorption of calcium in the small intestine depends upon the presence of vitamin D.

If your diet is deficient in calcium, it is leached from your bone stores, which increases your future risk of osteoporosis (brittle bones). Good intakes are especially important during childhood and adolescence, when bones are developing, and in later years when bones naturally start to thin (partly due to lower levels of the sex hormones oestrogen and testosterone).

Good intakes of calcium are vital throughout life for the growth, development and maintenance of strong, healthy bones and teeth. Calcium also plays a vital role in muscle contraction, nerve conduction, blood clotting, energy production and the regulation of many important metabolic enzymes.

Dietary sources of calcium

Calcium is found in milk (skimmed milk provides as much calcium as whole milk but without the additional fat); dairy products such as cheese, yogurt and fromage frais (but not butter); green leafy vegetables (especially broccoli but not spinach, whose oxalate content reduces its bioavailability); tinned salmon (including the bones); nuts and seeds; pulses; bread made from fortified flour, and eggs.

Overall, less than 40 per cent of dietary calcium from other sources is absorbed from the gut. Some types of dietary fibre (especially wheat phytates from unleavened bread) bind calcium in the bowel to form an insoluble, non-absorbable salt.

Drinking a pint of skimmed or semi-skimmed milk per day provides 720 mg calcium – almost your full daily requirement – in the readily absorbed form of calcium lactate.

The bioavailability of calcium in brassica vegetables (e.g. cabbage, cauliflower, broccoli, Brussels sprouts, swede) is unusually high (61 per cent, compared with 32 per cent for milk), for reasons that are not fully understood.

Deficiency

When dietary calcium is in short supply, it is leached from the bones to maintain heart muscle contraction. Low intakes of calcium are linked with wide-ranging symptoms affecting the muscles, bones and teeth. These include muscle aches, pains, twitching and cramps, heart palpitations, high blood pressure, osteoporosis, gum disease and loss of teeth.

Toxicity

An excess of calcium can cause lethargy, confusion and even coma. People with a tendency towards kidney stones should ideally take calcium supplements together with essential fatty acids, but are advised to seek medical advice first.

Chloride

Chloride is a negatively charged electrolyte of chlorine. It is widely present in the diet as salts of sodium, potassium and calcium. Together with sodium (outside cells) and potassium (inside cells), chloride ions are involved in the regulation of your body's fluid, electrolyte and acid/alkaline balance. It is also used to produce hydrochloric acid in the stomach.

Dietary sources of chloride

Chloride ions are present in just about every food, especially fruit; vegetables; seafood; seaweeds such as kelp; table salt and processed foods.

Deficiency

As chloride is widespread in foods, deficiency is uncommon except during periods of excessive vomiting. Excess intakes are more of a problem but during normal health, the body maintains a consistent blood level by excreting excess in sweat, urine and faeces.

Chromium

Chromium is a metallic trace element that exists in a number of oxidation states. While the hexavalent form of chromium (Cr^{6+}) used in industry and shiny car bumpers is highly toxic, the trivalent form of chromium (Cr^{3+}) is nutritionally essential. Trivalent chromium plays an important role in glucose control by regulating the interaction between insulin and receptors present in muscle and fat cells. It appears to do this in the form of a complex known as Glucose Tolerance Factor (GTF), which has been extracted from yeast. Although it has not been fully characterized (due to its instability), researchers suggest that GTF increases insulin binding to cells as well as the number of insulin receptors present on muscle and fat cells.

Dietary sources of chromium

As plants do not use chromium, their content depends on the amount and type of chromium present in the soil in which they are grown, and is highly variable. Potential sources include egg yolk; red meat; wholegrains; pulses; condiments such as black pepper and thyme; cheese; yeast; honey; fruit and vegetables.

Deficiency

Intestinal absorption is low (less than 2 per cent) except where chromium is present in the form of GTF such as that found in yeast. Low levels of chromium have been linked with poor glucose tolerance, weight loss and abnormal nerve function. A dietary lack of chromium appears to be a risk factor for Type 2 diabetes in some people.

Copper

Copper is a metallic trace element that is essential for healthy liver, brain and muscle function. Copper is a component of many anti-oxidant enzymes, including copper-zinc superoxide dismutase. It is involved in cholesterol, glucose and vitamin C metabolism, the production of brain chemicals and the manufacture of the tanning pigment, melanin, and the red blood pigment, haemoglobin. It is needed for the synthesis of collagen and is therefore involved in maintaining healthy bones, cartilage, hair and skin.

Dietary sources of copper

Rich sources include crustaceans, e.g. prawns; shellfish; offal; nuts; olives; pulses; wholegrain cereals and green vegetables.

Vegetable sources depend on the copper content of the soils in which they are grown.

Up to 70 per cent of dietary intake remains unabsorbed because it is bound to other bowel contents.

Deficiency

Lack of copper can occur in some conditions such as Crohn's or coeliac disease in which general nutrient absorption is reduced, and in people with a hereditary inability to process copper properly. Copper deficiency mainly affects the cardiovascular system and is associated with anaemia, low white-cell count, increased susceptibility to infection, fluid retention, loss of taste sensation, raised blood cholesterol levels and heart failure. It has also been linked with abnormal structure and pigmentation of skin and hair, osteoporosis and joint pains.

The risk of copper deficiency is greater when zinc intakes are high as the two interact to reduce copper's bioavailability. The ideal ratio of copper to zinc in both the diet and food supplements is 1:10.

Toxicity

Excess copper (for example, from drinking water supplied through copper pipes) is toxic at relatively low levels – just twice as high as normal intakes – causing restlessness, nausea, vomiting, colic and diarrhoea. Long-term high intakes can lead to copper-induced cirrhosis of the liver and brain damage.

Fluoride

Fluoride is a mineral that binds to bone to produce calcium fluoroapatite, which, in low concentrations, is more resistant to reabsorption than normal bone hydroxyapatite which may protect against osteoporosis (brittle bones). Similarly, it can strengthen tooth enamel so that it is more resistant to decay.

Dietary sources of fluoride

These include tea leaves (which provide 70 per cent of average intakes); fluorinated water supplies; seafood (especially oysters); pulses and wholegrains.

No EU RDA is currently set for fluoride. Intakes of between 1.5 mg and 4 mg have been suggested as desirable. Fluorination of drinking water provides between 1 mg and 3 mg fluoride a day.

Deficiency

Lack of fluoride is associated with weakened teeth and bones, leading to an increased risk of tooth decay and osteoporosis. Paradoxically, excess fluoride also promotes formation of abnormal, weakened bone and discoloured teeth (fluorosis) due to the presence of too much calcium fluoroapatite.

Iodine

Iodine is a non-metallic trace element that is essential for the production of two thyroid hormones, thyroxine and tri-iodothyronine. These regulate the basal metabolic rate – the speed at which energy and heat are produced in the body.

Dietary sources of iodine

These include marine fish; seafood; seaweed; iodized salt; milk from cattle receiving iodized feed; crops and cattle reared on soils exposed to sea spray.

Deficiency

Lack of iodine during pregnancy affects fetal brain development, leading to severe mental retardation (cretinism). Although this is uncommon in developed countries, it is a serious problem in some parts of the world, especially Indonesia. In endemic areas, this devastating condition can easily be prevented by administering injections of iodized oil to expectant mothers before the sixth month of pregnancy – preferably during the preconceptual period.

In adults, gross iodine deficiency leads to swelling of the thyroid gland (goitre).

Other symptoms that have been linked with iodine deficiency include an underactive thyroid gland, with associated symptoms of tiredness, lack of energy, weight gain, muscle weakness and susceptibility to cold.

Selenium plays a role in the metabolism of thyroid hormones, and the effects of iodine deficiency are made worse by low selenium intakes.

Toxicity

Up to 3 per cent of people are allergic to concentrated iodine solutions that are applied to disinfect the skin (for example, before a surgical operation). Excess iodine can cause a metallic taste in the mouth, oral sores, headache, diarrhoea, vomiting, rash and – as with a deficiency – can also lead to thyroid swelling (goitre).

Iron

Iron is an essential metallic mineral needed for production of the red blood pigment, haemoglobin and the red muscle pigment, myoglobin, both of which act as oxygen carriers. Two-thirds of your iron stores are circulating within the haemoglobin of your blood. Many enzyme systems, including cytochrome enzymes in the liver, also rely on iron for the production of energy, liver detoxification and immunity.

Dietary sources of iron

Rich sources include red meat; offal; shellfish; fish, especially sardines; wheatgerm; egg yolk; green vegetables; prunes and other dried fruit; fortified flour and cereals.

Dietary iron is available bound to protein as haem (from animal sources) and as inorganic salts. Absorption of haem iron is three times more efficient than that of non-haem iron, although most dietary iron is obtained in inorganic form. The presence of vitamin C in food increases absorption of inorganic iron by converting ferric iron (Fe^{3+}) to ferrous iron (Fe^{2+}). It's important to know, however, that over-boiling vegetables decreases their iron availability by up to 20 per cent.

Deficiency

Dietary iron intakes are falling due to decreased meat consumption and reduced energy intake. As a result, iron-deficiency anaemia (IDA) is increasingly common. The most vulnerable groups include infants over the age of six months (and younger ones if exclusively breastfed), toddlers, adolescents, menstruating or pregnant women and the elderly. Vegetarians and people who have high intakes of iron-absorption inhibitors (such as phytates) are also at risk.

Lack of iron quickly leads to the production of red blood cells that are much smaller and paler (due to lack of haemoglobin) than normal. This results in iron-deficiency anaemia, with symptoms of paleness, fast pulse, tiredness, exhaustion, dizziness, headache and even shortness of breath and angina if anaemia is severe.

Other symptoms that can occur in iron deficiency include generalized skin itching, concave brittle nails, hair loss, sore tongue, cracking at the corners of the mouth, reduced appetite and difficulty in swallowing.

Worldwide, iron deficiency is the most common nutritional disease, with most cases going unrecognized. Women are more at risk of iron deficiency than men because of blood loss during menstruation. This can result in a low-grade iron deficiency that is enough to impair immunity, without causing frank iron-deficiency anaemia. If anaemia is suspected, it is important to seek medical advice before taking iron supplements, as the cause needs to be determined. Iron supplements may mask iron deficiency by correcting changes usually seen in blood tests, so that a condition such as a bowel cancer (which can cause continuous tiny losses of blood) may initially be missed.

Toxicity

Your body has no specific mechanism for excreting excess iron. High intakes accumulate in the liver as storage proteins (haemosiderin, ferritin). Excess iron intakes can cause severe intestinal damage, as well as nausea, indigestion, constipation and bloody stools. It can also lead to liver damage, shock and coma. Excess is especially dangerous for children.

HAEMOCHROMATOSIS

Haemochromatosis is an autosomal recessive genetic condition in which the absorption of dietary iron is unregulated. Excess accumulation of iron can lead to liver cirrhosis, liver carcinoma, diabetes and heart failure. In Caucasian populations, haemochromatosis affects one in 140 people. In addition, one in 100 carries a genetic mutation that also increases the risk of iron accumulation. Another one in seven people carry one copy of the defective gene and have mildly increased iron stores, although significant iron loading is rare.

Magnesium

Magnesium is a metallic mineral needed as a cofactor for the function of over 300 enzymes. Few enzymes can work without it, and it is involved in every major metabolic reaction in the body, including the synthesis of protein and genetic material; metabolism of essential fatty acids and glucose; interactions between sex hormones and nuclear receptors; the production of brain chemicals and regulation of mood.

Magnesium is also vital for the integrity of ion pumps in cell membranes, which control the flow of sodium, potassium, calcium and chloride in and out of cells. This maintains the electrical potential across cell membranes that allows for nerve transmission, brain function and a regular heartbeat.

Seventy per cent of your body stores of magnesium are in your bones and teeth.

Dietary sources of magnesium

Rich sources include seafood; seaweed; meat; eggs; dairy products; wholegrains; pulses, especially soybeans; nuts; bananas; dark green leafy vegetables; chocolate and yeast.

Deficiency

People who are physically active can lose large amounts of magnesium in sweat. As magnesium is essential for the normal function of the parathyroid gland and for vitamin D metabolism, lack of magnesium markedly disturbs calcium balance and can lead to low calcium levels with muscle cramps. Deficiency has been implicated in constipation-predominant irritable bowel syndrome, migraine and hypertension.

Magnesium supplements above a dose of around 400 mg per day can cause diarrhoea by attracting water into the bowel. This can be beneficial, of course, and magnesium salts are used medicinally as a laxative.

Manganese

Manganese is a metallic element needed for the function of metalloenzymes involved in the synthesis of amino acids, carbohydrates, sex hormones, blood-clotting factors, cholesterol and some brain neurotransmitters. It is needed for the normal growth and development of bone, cartilage, collagen and structural molecules known as mucopolysaccharides. It also acts as an antioxidant.

Dietary sources of manganese

Sources include tea (1 mg per cup, on average); wholegrains; nuts and seeds; fruit; eggs; green leafy vegetables/herbs; offal; shellfish and milk.

Deficiency

The significance of manganese deficiency is currently unknown, but possible cases have been linked with reddening of black body hair, scaly skin, poor growth of hair and nails, disc and cartilage problems, poor blood clotting, glucose intolerance, poor memory and worsening intellect. It may also contribute to reduced fertility.

Toxicity

Industrial workers inhaling manganese dust (for example, during arc welding) have experienced neurological symptoms similar to Parkinson's disease (manganism), which remains an active issue in health and safety legislation.

Phosphorus

Phosphorus is a mineral that interacts with calcium to form calcium phosphate (hydroxyapatite) – the major structural component of bones and teeth. Most of your phosphorus is in your skeleton, but that remaining outside cells is vital for the production of energy-rich molecules (ATP, ADP), genetic material and for the activation of B vitamins involved in energy production. Vitamin D is essential for the absorption of phosphorus and calcium from the gut and for their deposition in bone.

Dietary sources of phosphorus

Phosphorus is widely found in foods such as fish; meat and poultry; eggs; dairy products; wholegrains; nuts; pulses; yeast extract and soft drinks such as colas.

Deficiency

Deficiency is unusual but can develop with long-term use of antacids containing aluminium hydroxide, which impairs phosphate absorption. Phosphorus deficiency symptoms include loss of appetite, anaemia, muscle weakness, bone pain, rickets and poor coordination.

High intakes can cause diarrhoea.

Potassium

Potassium is an alkaline metallic mineral that is concentrated inside body cells. Cells accumulate potassium by swapping it for sodium via sodium–potassium pumps found in all cell membranes. Potassium is essential for normal muscle contraction, including generation of a regular heartbeat, nerve conduction and glucose control. It is also involved in the production of genetic material, proteins and energy. The kidneys regulate blood potassium levels and keep them within a fairly narrow range.

A good intake of dietary potassium helps to flush excess sodium from the body via the kidneys to help lower a raised blood pressure.

Dietary sources of potassium

These include seafood; meat; fruit; vegetables; wholegrains; milk and dairy products; rock salt and low-sodium, potassium-enriched salt.

Deficiency

People taking certain diuretic drugs to reduce water retention may lose enough potassium to become deficient. Rarely, 'crash' or very strict diets can also lead to potassium deficiency, especially if little fruit or vegetables are eaten. Low intakes can cause rapid and irregular heartbeat, muscle weakness, irritability and may progress to nausea, vomiting, diarrhoea, low muscle tone and even paralysis.

Toxicity

The body usually maintains potassium levels within tight limits. Raised potassium levels (for example, due to kidney disease) can occur, causing heart failure, abnormal heart rhythms and cardiac arrest.

Selenium

Selenium is a metallic trace element that is so important to health that its incorporation into proteins (as selenocysteine, a recently identified amino acid) is directly controlled by your genes. Selenium is present in at least 30 human proteins (selenoenzymes) that are essential for cell growth, antioxidant protection, antibody synthesis and the activity of natural killer cells, which target virally infected cells and cancer cells. It is involved in the regulation of thyroid hormones and liver detoxification of cancer-causing chemicals (carcinogens). In parts of the world where selenium intakes are low, the incidence of cancer increases by two- to sixfold. Those with the lowest selenium intakes have the highest risk of developing leukaemia or cancers of the colon, rectum, breast, ovary, pancreas, prostate gland, bladder, skin and lungs.

Dietary sources of selenium

These include Brazil nuts (the richest dietary source); seafood; offal; meat (especially game); wholegrains; onions and garlic; broccoli, cabbage, mushrooms, radishes and celery and selenium-enriched yeast.

A healthy diet can no longer provide adequate intakes of selenium in many parts of Europe. Between 1975 and 1994, selenium intakes almost halved in the UK from 60 mcg to 34 mcg per day – mostly because the UK switched from using selenium-rich flour from the US and Canada to using flour produced in Europe.

Deficiency

Selenium is important for muscle cell function. In parts of China, selenium intakes are low enough to cause a form of heart failure (Keshan disease) and an unpleasant, deforming type of arthritis known as Kashin-Beck disease. These risks are even higher where intakes of other antioxidants such as vitamins A, C and E are also low. Symptoms and signs that have been linked to a lesser selenium deficiency include age spots, pale fingernail beds, increased susceptibility to viral infections (especially influenza) and some cancers.

Toxicity

Selenium toxicity can occur with intakes above 800 mcg daily, leading to a garlic odour on the breath, salivation, fragile or black fingernails, a metallic taste in the mouth, dizziness, nausea, vomiting and hair loss.

Silicon

Silicon is a non-metallic element that, in its pure form, is biologically inactive. As soluble silicate it is an essential trace element that strengthens collagen and elastin fibres and contributes to tissue elasticity. It increases mineralization of growing bones and is needed for the formation of cartilage.

Dietary sources of silicon

These include rice bran; wholegrains; green leafy vegetables; capsicum peppers; root vegetables; nuts and seeds.

There is no EU RDA for silicon. Intakes of 10 mg to 30 mg a day are believed to be adequate.

Deficiency

As the average diet supplies up to 50 mg per day from food and 10 mg per day from water, intakes are usually more than adequate. Silicon deficiency has been associated with bone and joint deformities and loss of bone mineralization (osteoporosis) in animals, but this has not been confirmed in humans.

Sodium

Sodium is a metallic mineral that is vital for regulating body-fluid balance. Most body sodium is present in tissue fluids as it is actively pumped out of cells in exchange for potassium ions. Sodium–potassium pumps in cell membranes transport three positively charged sodium ions out of a cell for every two positively charged potassium ions transported inside. This produces an electrical potential across cell membranes in which the inside of the cell is negatively charged compared with the outside. This electrical potential is vital for life, as it allows nerve and brain cells to conduct electrical signals and muscle cells to contract. In fact, the active transport of sodium and potassium ions in and out of body cells is one of the main energy-using processes contributing to your basal metabolic rate. It is estimated to account for 33 per cent of energy used by cells overall, and 70 per cent of energy used by nerve cells alone.

Dietary sources of sodium

These include table salt (sodium chloride); salted crisps; bacon; salted nuts; tinned products (especially those canned in brine); cured, smoked or pickled fish and meats, meat pastes and pâtés; ready-prepared meals; packet soups and sauces; stock cubes and yeast extract.

There is no EU RDA for sodium as most people take in too much. The UK reference nutrient intake for adults aged 19 to 50 years is 1,600 mg sodium (equivalent to 4 g salt) daily, and the average diet supplies 2,880 mg salt per day from food (not counting salt added during cooking or at the table). Variable amounts are obtained from drinking water, as sodium is added during softening of hard water. Soft water contains up to 25 mg sodium per litre, and hard water up to 75 mg per litre. Contamination of wellsprings with seawater can also affect its sodium content.

Toxicity

Excess sodium leads to fluid retention and high blood pressure in those who are sodium-sensitive. Toxicity leads to vomiting, muscle weakness, kidney damage and metabolic acidosis and can be lethal. Children are especially vulnerable.

Zinc

Zinc is a metallic element that acts as a cofactor for over 200 metabolic enzymes. It regulates the activity of genes in response to hormone triggers, playing an important role in growth, sexual maturity and wound healing. Zinc is also important for immune function.

Dietary sources of zinc

These include red meat; seafood, especially oysters; offal; wholegrains; pulses; eggs; cheese and yeast.

Deficiency

In some parts of the world, dietary zinc deficiency is common and results in growth retardation, physical and mental retardation in children, impaired nerve function, dermatitis, hair loss, diarrhoea, loss of appetite, taste and smell, anaemia, susceptibility to infections, delayed wound healing and macular degeneration. In males, zinc deficiency is associated with low testosterone levels, delayed male puberty, reduced male fertility and increased risk of prostatitis (inflammation of the prostate gland).

Toxicity

Excess can cause abdominal pain, nausea, vomiting, lethargy, anaemia and dizziness. Zinc affects iron and copper uptake when taken at doses greater than 50 mg per day. Zinc supplements often contain copper at a ratio of 10:1 (10 mg zinc to 1 mg copper).

6

Functional foods: phytochemicals and probiotics

As well as providing macronutrients, vitamins, minerals and fibre, fruit and vegetables provide other non-nutrient substances that have beneficial effects on human health. Although not deemed essential, these make an important contribution towards good health as they influence human metabolism in a positive way. So although you could survive without them, your risk of some long-term conditions such as atherosclerosis (hardening and fur-ring-up of the arteries), high blood pressure, raised cholesterol levels, heart disease, stroke and even cancer could be increased. These plant-based substances are known as phytochemicals (after the Greek word *phyton* meaning plant). As far as the plants are con-cerned, some of these phytochemicals provide colour to attract the organisms that help with their fertilization and dissemination (for example, purple anthocyanin pigments in blueberries), protection against the sun (red lycopene in tomatoes) or have an antimicro-bial action against plant viruses and other predators (flavonoids in apples). When these plants are eaten, phytochemicals contribute to flavour (the astringent tannins in tea and wine) and can also affect your body's metabolic functions. As they are not classed as macronutrients, vitamins or minerals, they deserve special atten-tion, together with probiotics – the so-called 'friendly' digestive bacteria that contribute to bowel health and immunity. One of the hottest debates in nutritional medicine currently centres around probiotics and the beneficial effects they have on human health.

Phytochemicals

More than 30,000 phytochemicals have been identified, which can be divided on the basis of their chemical structures into phenols, carotenoids, phytosterols and sulphur-containing compounds. The average diet is believed to supply more than 1 g of phytochemicals per day, which is good, but obviously people who eat the most plant-based foods (including tea drinkers) will obtain the greatest amounts and obtain the most benefits.

Phenols

Phenols are a group of plant chemicals that have two or more aromatic phenol rings in their structure. They contribute to the colour, taste and smell of many foods – capsaicinoids give chilli peppers their fiery hotness, for example, while limonenes produce both the orange-lemon scents of citrus fruit and the more pungent smell of fresh pine nuts. The amount present in fruit and vegetables depends on the cultivars (for example, whether you are eating a green Granny Smith or a rosy Pink Lady apple) and on their growing conditions, their ripeness and how they are processed and stored.

Phenols form a diverse group that includes tannins, lignans, stilbenes, phenolic acids and flavonoids, of which the latter are the best studied and understood.

Flavonoids (sometimes known as bioflavonoids) are antioxidants that protect plants from attack by microbes, insects and UV light.

According to researchers from Harvard University, there is a growing body of evidence that regular consumption of some flavonoids can have a marked effect on human health, for example by protecting against heart attacks. Among the most important flavonoids are the isoflavones, the catechins and the anthocyanins.

Isoflavones

Isoflavones have a similar structure to the human hormone oestrogen and are therefore classed as phytoestrogens (i.e. plant oestrogens). Other phytochemicals with an oestrogen-like action in the body include lignans (present in high concentrations in linseed/flax seed) and stilbenes (e.g. resveratrol found in the skin and pips of grapes and in wines, especially red wine, which tends to remain in contact with grape skins for longer during maceration). The role of these chemicals within the plants is not fully understood, but it has been suggested that their oestrogen-like properties may form part of the natural defences of some plants. In theory, they might lower male fertility in the herbivore species that eat them, and thereby reduce the number of animals who are actively seeking a snack! Whatever their role in plants, they have a physiological action in humans, and global consumption of phytoestrogens is increasing.

Of the thousand or more isoflavones that have been identified, five are present in significant amounts in the human diet: genistein, daidzein and glycitein are mainly derived from soy, while formononetin and biochanin A (which are metabolized to form daidzein and genistein) are obtained from chickpeas, lentils and mung beans. In cultures such as Japan, where soy is a dietary staple, intakes of isoflavones are between 50 mg and 100 mg per day, compared with typical Western intakes of just 2 mg to 5 mg isoflavones per day. As a result, blood levels of phytoestrogens in people following a traditional Japanese diet are as much as 110 times higher than those typically found in the West, and this is thought to account for the unusually low incidence of heart disease and breast cancer seen in those following a traditional Japanese diet.

Dietary isoflavones are mostly present in an inactive form (attached to sugars to form glycosides) such as genistin and daidzin. Once ingested, bacteria in your large intestines remove the sugar to release the active forms (isoflavone aglycones) such as genistein and daidzein. Some people possess good amounts of beneficial probiotic bacteria (such as lactobacilli, bifidobacteria) that further metabolize daidzein to a more powerful oestrogen called equol. Equol has a higher antioxidant activity than any other isoflavone, and those classed as 'equol producers' may gain greater health benefits from dietary isoflavones than 'non-equol producers'.

Isoflavones interact with human oestrogen receptors. Although this interaction is between 100 and 1,000 times weaker than that of human oestrogen itself, they occupy the receptors and block the access of the stronger human hormones. This can damp down potentially harmful, high oestrogen states (which have been associated with health problems such as breast cancer and endometriosis, for example). They also provide useful oestrogen activity when oestrogen levels are low after the female menopause, which may help to reduce oestrogen-withdrawal symptoms such as hot flushes and night sweats. On the other hand, some phytoestrogens are now recognized as endocrine disruptors, which may potentially interfere with reproductive health just like certain synthetic pesticides (for example, DDT), industrial lubricants (PCBs) and plasticizers (Bisphenol A). There is growing concern too from some nutritionists about the widespread use of isoflavone-rich infant soy formulas. In some countries, such as the UK, Australia and New Zealand, soy-based formulas are now mainly reserved for infants who do not tolerate those based on cows' milk proteins. Women who are pregnant, breastfeeding or planning for a baby should probably also use soy foods with caution, but for older people at risk of heart disease, a soy-rich diet may offer some benefits, as follows.

Isoflavones and heart disease

Japanese people who eat a traditional soy-rich diet have one of the lowest rates of coronary heart disease in the world. Their high isoflavone intake is suggested as one explanation due to a variety of mechanisms, including their antioxidant action and their ability to interact with oestrogen receptors to promote arterial dilation and reduce blood pressure, cholesterol levels and abnormal platelet clumping. A meta-analysis of 23 trials, for example, found beneficial reductions in total cholesterol, LDL-cholesterol and triglycerides, with increased beneficial HDL-cholesterol. The evidence of benefit was so strong that, in 1999, the US Food and Drug Administration (FDA) approved the use of a health claim that daily consumption of 25 g soy protein − in a diet that is low in saturated fat and cholesterol − may reduce the risk of heart disease. This advice still stands. The European Food Safety Authority took a much more rigorous view, however, and rejected this scientific claim, stating that a cause-and-effect relationship had not yet been established between the consumption of soy protein and the reduction of LDL-cholesterol concentrations. (The EFSA also rejected a claim that regular consumption of large amounts of water can reduce the risk of dehydration, which illustrates just how rigorous their approach can be!) But a recent medical review looking at the pros and cons of phytoestrogens suggested that 'people at risk of heart disease may want to consider replacing at least a portion of their meat intake with soy'.

Isoflavones and cancer

Because they block the interaction of stronger human oestrogens with their tissue receptors, isoflavones may protect against oestrogen-sensitive cancers of the breast and, in males, of the prostate gland. This is supported by a number of observational trials in which those eating the most soy are considerably less likely to have a high risk of breast or prostate cancer than those eating the least. A study published in the *Journal of the National Cancer Institute* involving 21,852 Japanese women, for example, found that those with the highest consumption of isoflavones were 54 per cent less likely to develop breast cancer than those with the lowest intake. This remained true even after adjusting for reproductive history, family history, smoking and other dietary factors. Another study published in the *British Journal of Cancer*, involving 35,000 women, found an 18 per cent reduced risk of breast cancer relative to those consuming the least intake of isoflavones. In both studies, the protection was highest in post-menopausal women. However, observational studies can only show an association – they do not provide definite proof.

Not surprisingly, there has been concern over a possible detrimental effect of isoflavone supplements in women with pre-existing breast cancer due to their oestrogen-like action. A critical review of the literature concluded that, overall, there is no impressive data suggesting that adult consumption of soy/isoflavones affects the risk of developing breast cancer, or that soy consumption affects the survival of breast-cancer patients. This has now been substantiated by the American Institute for Cancer Research (AICR) who recently stated that breast cancer patients and survivors no longer need to worry about eating moderate amounts of soy foods. Different doctors have different opinions, however, so seek advice from your own doctor.

Isoflavones and menopause

Phytoestrogens have a weak oestrogen-like action that may reduce the oestrogen-withdrawal symptoms associated with the female menopause. This may explain why the prevalence of hot flushes among Asian women is generally lower (10 per cent to 20 per cent) than is observed in most Western populations (70 per cent to 80 per cent).

The use of hormone-replacement therapy (HRT) has fallen out of favour due to fears that its use may increase the risk of breast cancer, so women are turning more and more to natural treatments such as isoflavone supplements. Although results from different trials have varied, and there is a large placebo effect, a recent systematic review and meta-analysis of the results from 19 randomized controlled trials found that isoflavone extracts reduced hot flushes by 39 per cent compared with placebo. Even though the overall combined results showed a significant tendency in favour of soy, the authors still stated that it was difficult to establish conclusive results given the highly variable results from different studies. This may be explained in part by the suggestion that only women who are equol producers will derive meaningful benefit.

INCREASING YOUR NATURAL INTAKE OF PHYTOESTROGENS

Aim to consume more of the following foods:

Beans, especially chickpeas, lentils, alfalfa and mung beans, soybeans and soy products (e.g. tofu marinated in low-salt soy sauce)

Vegetables, dark green leafy vegetables (e.g. broccoli, spinach, cabbage) and exotic members of the cruciferous family (e.g. Chinese leaves, kohl rabi), celery, fennel

Nuts, almonds, cashew nuts, hazelnuts, peanuts, walnuts and cold-pressed nut oils

Seeds, especially flaxseed, pumpkin, sesame, sunflower and sprouted seeds

Wholegrains, especially corn, buckwheat, millet, oats, rye and wheat

Fresh fruit, including apples, avocados, bananas, mangoes, papayas and rhubarb

Dried fruit, especially dates, figs, prunes and raisins

Herbs, especially angelica, chervil, garlic, ginger, parsley, rosemary and sage

Catechins

Tea leaves are the richest dietary source of a group of antioxidants known as catechins. As tea is the second most common drink in the world after water, those who regularly drink green, white or black tea obtain sizeable intakes of these beneficial catechins. Other dietary sources include apples, pears, berries and dark chocolate.

Tea is prepared from the young leaves and leaf buds of an Asian shrub, *Camellia sinensis*. Green tea is made by steaming and drying the fresh tea leaves immediately after harvesting, while black tea is made by crushing and fermenting the freshly cut tea leaves so that they oxidize before drying. This allows natural enzymes in the tea leaves to produce the characteristic red-brown colour and reduced astringency. White tea is similar to green tea in that it is not fermented, but is only made from new tea buds, picked before they open. These have a white appearance due to the presence of fine silvery hairs.

DID YOU KNOW?

White tea contains around 15 mg caffeine per cup, compared to 20 mg for green tea and 40 mg for black tea.

A third of the dry weight of tea leaves consists of antioxidants, with green tea containing more catechins and black tea containing more complex theaflavins and thearubigins which, although originally thought to be less beneficial, are now known to have similar antioxidant power. Black tea, as brewed in the UK, contains around 200 mg flavonoids per cup. Although it has been suggested that adding milk to a cup of tea might blunt its antioxidant capacity, a number of studies have now found that milk is unlikely to reduce the bioavailability of tea flavonoids.

Tea and heart disease

Consumption of tea flavonoids increases the antioxidant capacity of blood, and has been shown to improve blood-vessel reactivity (so that blood vessels are able to dilate more readily, as needed) and blood flow through the coronary arteries. This might be expected to provide some protection against heart attack. A review published in the *European Journal of Clinical Nutrition* found clear evidence for a protective effect of black tea against coronary heart disease at an intake of at least three cups per day. A meta-analysis of 13 studies published in the *American Journal of Clinical Nutrition* concluded that for every cup of green tea you consume each day, your risk of developing coronary heart disease is reduced by another 10 per cent. Perhaps surprisingly, they did not find a protective effect from drinking black tea, and more research is obviously needed.

Tea and metabolism

Catechins can boost your basal metabolic rate by inhibiting a metabolic enzyme (catechol-0-methyl transferase) that breaks down a neurotransmitter called noradrenaline. A rise in noradrenaline levels stimulates the amount of energy burned in body cells (thermogenesis). Tea extracts may also block the activity of intestinal enzymes (gastric and pancreatic lipases) needed to digest dietary fat, so that less fat is absorbed. Research also suggests that drinking tea can have beneficial effects on metabolism to suppress the high blood glucose levels and insulin resistance associated with diabetes, as well as reducing weight gain. These effects are still under investigation in humans, but a study of 300 elderly people living in Cyprus found that drinking one to two cups per day for at least 30 years was associated with a 70 per cent lower odds of developing Type 2 diabetes, even after adjusting for other factors such as age, weight, smoking, activity level and dietary habits.

Although the jury may still be out, if you enjoy a cup of tea then carry on drinking it – in fact, aim for at least two or three cups per day!

Anthocyanins

Anthocyanins are the water-soluble pigments that give many fruit, vegetables and flowers their lovely red, blue or purple colour. They are also responsible for the red coloration of autumn leaves. The colour of anthocyanins depends on the level of acidity present, and these pigments are often used as pH indicators (red = acid, blue = alkali) such as the famous litmus test based on a blend of dyes extracted from lichens. Within plants, anthocyanins act as a 'sunscreen' by absorbing blue-green and UV light, and also have antimicrobial actions to protect plants against infection.

FANCY A PURPLE TOMATO?

Scientists recently developed a genetically modified purple tomato by inserting two snapdragon genes. These genes switch on a tomato gene that regulates the synthesis of tomato anthocyanins so that the purple colour is 'natural' to the tomato plant and is not owed to a flower pigment that is not normally present in tomatoes.

Different plants contain different types of anthocyanin (e.g. cyanidin, delphinidin, malvidin, pelargonidin, peonidin, petunidin, myrtilin) and over 630 have now been identified in nature. Many of these are in the food we eat, and intakes are estimated at 23 mg per day in Europe and 650 mg per day in North America (partly accounted for by a particular love of bilberries). A serving of 100 g berries provides up to 500 mg of anthocyanins.

Numerous studies show that the anthocyanins you eat can have a wide range of biological actions in the body. They are highly antioxidant and can have effects that vary from reducing blood pressure, abnormal platelet clotting, glucose intolerance and cholesterol levels to reducing inflammation and protecting against coronary heart disease. As well as having an antioxidant action, they may act as biological response modifiers by switching off genes involved in abnormal cell proliferation and the growth of abnormal blood vessels (angiogenesis), which together may reduce the risk of cancer. These beneficial effects are undoubtedly part of the reason why high intakes of fruit and vegetables are so beneficial to health – and possibly why a rosy red apple a day might help keep the doctor away!

Carotenoids

At the other end of the colour scale, carotenoids are antioxidant plant pigments found in yellow, orange and dark green fruits and vegetables, including sweetcorn, carrots, pumpkins, mangoes, oranges, peaches, guavas, watermelons, spinach and other dark green leafy vegetables. A few carotenoids are red, such as the lycopene found in tomatoes, and astaxanthin – the red carotenoid pigment found in certain algae which, when consumed by flamingos, turns their plumage such a glorious shade of pink.

Over 600 carotenoids have been identified, of which around 50 can be converted into vitamin A in the body and are said to have provitamin A activity. This is inefficient, however, and it takes 6 mcg of betacarotene (one of the most common carotenoids) to yield 1 mcg of retinol vitamin A. For other carotenoids with provitamin A activity, twice as much is needed (12 mcg) to yield 1 mcg retinol. A carrot weighing 100 g contains around 2,400 mcg of betacarotene, for example, which if you divide by six is equivalent to 400 mcg of retinol. In contrast, 100 g of calf's liver provides around 25,200 mcg of retinol vitamin A.

Some carotenoids without provitamin A activity are also important for human health, most notably astaxanthin, lycopene, lutein and zeaxanthin.

TURNING ORANGE

Eating excessive amounts of carotenes – for example, from carrot juice – can lead to carotenodermia, in which the skin acquires an orange colour that resembles cheap fake tan. This is considered harmless, and quickly resolves once intakes are reduced. Excessive intakes of retinol vitamin A, however, are highly toxic, as discussed in Chapter 4.

Astaxanthin

As mentioned above, astaxanthin is a carotenoid produced by some red yeasts and microalgae to provide protection against ultraviolet light. High concentrations are found in a tropical alga, *Haematococcus pluvialis*, which remains green until exposed to strong sunlight, when it produces astaxanthin and turns red. When Antarctic krill, prawns, salmon, rainbow trout and crabs eat red microalgae, the astaxanthin becomes concentrated in their flesh, roes or shells, which acquire a pink colour. If you regularly consume krill-oil supplements or crustacea, therefore, you will obtain significant amounts of astaxanthin in your diet. Research into the effects of astaxanthin on human health is in its infancy. However, a number of recent reviews, including one in the *American Journal of Cardiology*, discuss its potential for beneficial effects on your antioxidant levels, cholesterol balance, arterial blood flow and coronary heart disease, as well as for visual acuity.

> ## WHY FARMED FISH AND EGGS LOOK SO GOOD
>
> Astaxanthin is added to some animal feeds to colour farm-raised salmon and to intensify the colour of hens' egg yolks. And do you know why lobster shells turn from blue to red when cooked? It's because heating releases astaxanthin from the proteins to which it is bound.

Lycopene

Lycopene is a red pigment found in tomatoes, pink guava, papaya, red/pink grapefruit and watermelon. When cooked, tomatoes release five times more lycopene than is available from raw tomatoes, so concentrated products such as tomato ketchup, tomato purée, passata – and pizzas – are among the richest dietary sources of lycopene. At last – a nutritional reason for fully enjoying a juicy Margharita pizza! Like other carotenoids, lycopene is fat-soluble, so drizzling healthy olive or rapeseed oils over your pizza slice, in true Mediterranean fashion, increases your dietary absorption of lycopene as much as threefold. Why is lycopene so good for you? Because evidence is accumulating that it protects against both coronary heart disease and cancer – the two biggest killers in the developed world.

Lycopene and coronary heart disease

People who regularly eat tomatoes and tomato products are 30 to 47 per cent less likely to develop heart disease than those who eat them infrequently. Lycopene is the most likely protective factor. A recent meta-analysis of 12 studies show that it has a marked cholesterol-lowering action – taking 25 mg supplements daily can reduce cholesterol levels by 10 per cent which, as the authors point out, is comparable to the effect of low-dose statin drugs. In addition, the studies showed that lycopene supplements noticeably reduced systolic blood pressure by, on average, 5.6 mmHg (an effect equivalent to some prescribed anti-hypertensive medications).

Lycopene and cancer

People with the highest dietary intakes of lycopene have the lowest incidence of certain cancers, especially those of the mouth, oesophagus, stomach, lung, colon, rectum, cervix and prostate gland. Although it is possible that lycopene may just act as a biomarker for tomato consumption, and that other phytochemicals present in tomatoes (such as phytoene, phytofluene, quercetin, kaempferol, naringenin) are also involved, cell studies in the laboratory confirm that lycopene has a number of powerful anti-tumour effects in addition to its antioxidant action. In particular, it inhibits growth factors and cell-membrane proteins involved in the spread and invasion of cancer cells. Follow-up studies involving more than 48,000 male health professionals found that men who ate more than ten servings of tomato products per week were 35 per cent less likely to develop prostate cancer than those eating less than 1.5 servings per week. And, after accounting for smoking, people with the lowest levels of lycopene are three times more likely to develop lung cancer than those with the highest intakes. Of course, it's possible that people who eat lots of tomatoes and lycopene generally select a healthy diet and make other healthy lifestyle choices such as not smoking, exercising regularly and avoiding excess alcohol. But no similar associations have been found for other carotenoids associated with a healthy diet, such as betacarotene, alphacarotene, lutein or beta-crypto-xanthin. So while you may not want to take lycopene supplements, it's certainly worth eating more cooked tomatoes and indulging in the odd splash of tomato ketchup and the occasional slice of pizza. Drizzled with olive oil, of course!

Lutein

Lutein is a bright yellow pigment found in yellow-orange fruits and vegetables. It's also abundant (though disguised by the green pigment, chlorophyll) in dark green leaves such as kale or spinach, and contributes to the colour of egg yolks.

Lutein is important for vision. It is preferentially concentrated within the macula – the part of the retina responsible for fine sight such as recognizing faces and reading this print. Within the macula, lutein is partly converted into another carotenoid called zeaxanthin. Both lutein and zeaxanthin protect the macula by filtering out harmful, visible blue light, and through their anti-oxidant action, which neutralizes damaging free radicals generated during the chemical processes involved in light detection.

As lutein cannot be made in the body, good dietary intakes are vital for eye health. Lack of lutein causes depletion of macular pigment and increases the risk of age-related macular degeneration – one of the leading causes of registered blindness in people over the age of 50 years. Age-related macular degeneration is a particularly distressing and isolating condition as it produces visual distortion followed by 'blanking' out of faces and print so you can't read. There are two types of AMD: 'wet' in which new, fragile blood vessels leak fluid into surrounding tissues, and 'dry' where new blood-vessel formation has not occurred. Wet AMD is treated with laser therapy to seal leaking blood vessels and, increasingly, with drugs injected into the eye. For dry AMD, however, the mainstay of treatment – and prevention – is to obtain a good dietary intake of lutein-rich foods. A number of studies have found an inverse relationship between dietary lutein/zeaxanthin intakes and advanced AMD that is statistically important. People with macular degeneration have, on average, 70 per cent less lutein and zeaxanthin in their eyes than those with healthy vision, while good intakes of lutein and zeaxanthin are associated with a reduced risk of age-related macular degeneration of up to 40 per cent.

The LAST study (Lutein Antioxidant Supplementation Trial) showed that macular pigment optical density increased over time in those taking 10 mg lutein supplements daily for one year, and declined slightly without supplementation. Visual acuity also improved in those with 'dry' AMD by the equivalent of 5.4 letters on a Snellen chart with improved contrast sensitivity. No improvement occurred in those taking inactive placebo. In the follow-up LAST2 study, individuals with the lowest macular pigment optical density, and in greatest need of supplements, were most likely to benefit from either a 10 mg lutein supplement or a lutein plus antioxidant supplement. For those responding, macular pigment optical density continued to increase for at least 12 months, with the benefits still continuing when the trial ended. Diet should always come first, of course, but where people are unwilling, or unable, to eat more lutein-rich fruit and vegetables, there is a strong argument for proposing a lutein supplement as a safety net to augment the diet. The potential benefits for eye health greatly outweigh any risks, which are negligible.

Phytosterols

Phytosterols (also known as plant sterols) such as sitosterol, stigmasterol and campesterol are the third main category of phytochemicals as mentioned at the beginning of this chapter. They have a similar structure to the cholesterol found in animals and, as a result, can block cholesterol absorption from the intestines although they are not much absorbed themselves. As well as reducing uptake of the cholesterol you eat in animal-based foods, they also block absorption of the cholesterol made in your liver, which is squirted into your gut within bile. As the blocked cholesterol is voided from your bowels (along with most of the plant sterols), your circulating cholesterol levels are reduced if your diet contains these beneficial phytochemicals.

A large trial involving over 22,500 men and women living in Norfolk in the UK showed that people with the highest dietary intake of plant sterols have the lowest cholesterol levels. Another study showed that a sterol-rich diet can reduce levels of harmful LDL-cholesterol by around 15 per cent – enough to lower considerably your risk of a heart attack or stroke. Plant sterols work in a different way to the statin drugs prescribed to lower elevated cholesterol levels and which have a direct effect on the liver. The two can therefore be used together for a synergistic effect. Research from the Mayo Clinic demonstrates that adding plant sterols to statin medication has been shown to reduce cholesterol levels even more than by doubling the statin dose.

The richest sources of plant sterols are vegetable oils, wholegrains and nuts. The average diet provides around 400 mg sterols per day, although some vegetarians may obtain three times as much. For optimum cholesterol-lowering benefits, however, an intake of 2 g per day is ideal. Higher doses do not appear to enhance their effectiveness, and may reduce absorption of some dietary carotenoids (although this is easily overcome by eating an additional serving of a carotenoid-rich fruit or vegetable per day – something we should be aiming to do anyway!).

While diet should always come first, it is difficult to obtain optimum amounts of sterols from normal food sources alone, especially as the phytosterols within plants are naturally bound to fibre, which limits their action. Fortified products (yogurt, spreads, milk and dairy-free drinks) have therefore been developed to augment dietary intakes.

Sulphur-containing compounds

Sulphur-containing plant chemicals are the fourth main category of phytochemicals to consider. We mainly obtain these in the form of sulphides (from the onion or Allium family of plants, which includes garlic, shallots, leeks and chives) and glucosino-lates (from the Brassica or cabbage family).

Sulphides

Garlic is a source of the powerful sulphur-containing antioxidant allicin, whose full chemical name is diallyl thiosulphinate. Allicin is formed from an odourless precursor, alliin, which is an amino acid unique to the garlic family. Alliin is stored within garlic cells, separated from the enzyme, alliinase, that breaks it down. It is only when garlic is crushed or cut that alliin and alliinase come together to produce allicin with its characteristic odour. Fresh garlic can contain up to 4 g of alliin per kilogram, but if garlic is cooked immediately after peeling, alliinase is inactivated and some of its benefits are lost. Thus the best way to preserve the maximum benefit from garlic cloves in your cooking is to add them right at the end, rather than at the beginning as is more usual. This will increase the pungency of any odours you give off afterwards, however – great for keeping away vampires, not so good when it comes to attracting new friends.

Garlic and cholesterol

Some, but not all studies have found that garlic tablets can lower circulating cholesterol levels with proposed mech-anisms including reduced cholesterol production in the liver and increased excretion of fatty acids. Discrepancies may relate to differences in the garlic preparations used, the dose and the duration of the trial. A meta-analysis of data from 29 trials, published in 2009, found that garlic did reduce total choles-terol levels by 19 per cent and triglycerides by 11 per cent, although there were no relative changes in LDL- or HDL-cholesterol balance.

Garlic and blood pressure

Sulphur compounds formed from the breakdown of allicin have also been found to react with red blood cells to produce hydrogen sulphide, which relaxes blood vessels. This can promote circulation through small arteries (arterioles) and small veins (venules) as well as lowering blood pressure in those with an elevated systolic blood pressure. A meta-analysis of data from ten trials found that, compared with inactive placebo, garlic extracts reduced blood pressure by 16.3/9.3 mmHg in people with hypertension, which is better than is achieved with many prescribed drugs! Interestingly, it did not markedly affect blood pressure in those without hypertension (which is important to reduce potential side effects such as faintness), and research is currently under way to work out why.

Garlic and cancer

The strongest evidence for benefit from garlic constituents is in the area of cancer protection. The sulphurous compounds found in garlic have been shown to suppress the formation of carcinogenic substances (nitrosamines) in the body, and to arrest the growth of human cancer cells either through effects on the cell life cycle or by a direct interaction with DNA. Although most of these effects were observed at concentrations higher than those encountered in the normal diet, a recent meta-analysis of 21 studies involving over 543,000 people suggested that those eating the largest amount of Allium vegetables were 46 per cent less likely to develop stomach cancer than those with the lowest intake. There was a definite dose-response effect, so that every 20 g of Allium vegetables consumed daily reduced the risk of gastric cancer by 9 per cent. However, other dietary factors not accounted for may have contributed to these effects and, for now, this remains an interesting finding that should encourage you to consume more French onion soup and to add as much garlic to your cooking as you can tolerate (but remember to put it in just at the end).

Glucosinolates

Glucosinolates are sulphur-containing compounds, derived from glucose and an amino acid, found mainly in brassica vegetables such as mustard, horseradish, Brussels sprouts, radish, turnip and cauliflower. When these plants are crushed, chopped or chewed, the glucosinolates are broken down by an enzyme (myrosinase) to release a number of hot or bitter products that discourage animals from eating them – though humans often find them tasty! These substances include isothiocyanates (mustard, horse-radish), bitter sinigrin (Brussels sprouts, cauliflower), thiocyanates and indoles. A study of intakes in Germany found that average consumptions of glucosinolates were around 14.5 mg per day.

Microbiological studies show that these glucosinolates have a notable antibacterial action and might be useful in reducing our susceptibility to intestinal infections.

Their most useful action, however, is in protecting against cancer. Those with the highest intake of glucosinolates – especially sulforaphane found in broccoli – have been shown, in epidemiological studies, to have a lower risk of developing cancers of the bowel (colon and rectum).

Currently there are no recommended dietary intakes for most phytochemicals except sterols for lowering cholesterol levels. However, eating a wide variety of fruit and vegetables as part of your five-a-day (minimum, preferably eight to ten a day) servings will provide good intakes. These phytochemicals are one of the key contributors to findings that people who eat the most fruit and vegetables are the least likely to develop cancer. A review of over 200 clinical studies found a consistent protective effect of fruit and vegetables against cancers of the stomach, oesophagus, lung, mouth and throat, uterus, pancreas and colon. The greatest protection came from eating raw vegetables, onions, garlic, carrots, green vegetables, members of the cabbage family and tomatoes – all of which are rich sources of phytochemicals, as discussed above. Similarly, a meta-analysis of eight studies involving over 257,000 people, published in *The Lancet*, found that eating three to five servings of fruit and vegetables per day reduced the risk of stroke by 11 per cent, compared with those eating fewer than three a day. However, those eating more than five a day had a 26 per cent lower risk. Overall, it seems that each additional portion of fruit you eat per day reduces your risk of stroke by 11 per cent, while each additional portion of vegetables reduces your risk by 3 per cent. And when it comes to heart disease, the results from studies involving over 278,000 people found that eating three to five servings of fruit and vegetables per day reduced the risk of coronary heart disease by 7 per cent compared to eating fewer than three servings a day. Those who ate more than five servings per day, however, enjoyed a 17 per cent lower risk.

The evidence is strong that, although eating five servings of fruit and vegetables per day is good, eating more than five is considerably better.

Probiotics

The term *probiotic* literally means 'for life' and is used to describe the 'friendly' bacteria and yeasts found in some fermented foods such as live 'bio' yogurts, fermented milk drinks and sauerkraut. According to the World Health Organization definition, probiotics are 'live microorganisms which, when administered in adequate amounts, confer a health benefit on the host'.

The most common probiotics are lactic-acid bacteria such as *Lactobacillus acidophilus*, *Bifidobacterium longum* and related strains.

Because these are acid-tolerant, a considerable number survive passage through the stomach and small intestines to reach your large bowel. As you open your bowels regularly, the most beneficial probiotic bacteria are those that attach to landing sites on the intestinal wall where they set up colonies to replenish their numbers.

Altogether, your gut contains around 11 trillion bacteria – more than the number of human cells in your body. Together, these bacteria weigh an astonishing 1.5 kg and provide a major contribution to the bulk of bowel motions. Every gram of fibre you eat, for example, increases the weight of faeces by 5 g as fibre fuels the growth of these bowel bacteria.

Ideally, at least 70 per cent of 'your' bacteria should be healthy probiotic bacteria, and only 30 per cent should be other bowel commensals (bacteria that live happily on or in another organism without causing harm) such as *E. coli*. In practice, however, the balance is usually the other way round.

Probiotic bacteria play an important role in maintaining digestive health by:

* producing lactic and acetic acids to discourage growth of other potentially harmful organisms
* secreting natural antibiotics known as bacteriocins to help discourage overgrowth of other less beneficial intestinal bacteria
* competing with harmful bacteria and yeasts for available nutrients
* competing with other bacteria for attachment sites on intestinal cell walls – literally crowding them out so they pass through the intestines without gaining a foothold
* stimulating your production of natural antiviral substances such as interferons
* helping to stimulate your immune defences against bacteria in general. A large part of your immune defences are present

within the wall of the ileum in the small intestines, where they form pale areas known as Peyer's patches (see Chapter 1).

As discussed above, probiotic bacteria also metabolize some of the phytoestrogens in your diet to release the more active plant oestrogen called equol, which has an oestrogen-like action. In addition, the probiotic bacteria (which produce lactic acid) produce short-chain fatty acids that act as a major energy source for your intestinal lining cells. These beneficial short-chain fatty acids are also absorbed from the colon and transported to your liver, where they have a positive effect on your cholesterol metabolism.

Lactic-acid bacteria can inhibit the growth of harmful bacteria that cause gastroenteritis such as *Bacillus cereus*, *Salmonella typhi*, *Shigella dysenteriae*, *Escherichia coli*, *Staphylococcus aureus* and *Clostridium difficile*. They can also reduce diarrhoea caused by taking antibiotics that lower the level of natural lactic-acid bacteria within the intestines. And, as alteration in normal bowel bacterial balance has been linked with irritable bowel syndrome (IBS), repopulating the bowel with lactic-acid bacteria can improve associated symptoms such as bloating, discomfort, constipation and diarrhoea. This is thought to result from their ability to reduce the presence of gas-producing enterobacteria that are associated with IBS symptoms.

Oral administration of lactic-acid bacteria has been shown to be safe in several hundred human clinical trials. Caution is needed, however, when considering their use in some immuno-compromised patients and in those with intestinal bleeding, although the lack of harmful effects from lactobacilli and bifido-bacteria appears to extend across all age groups, including immuno-compromised individuals.

Probiotics are immensely popular, and an estimated 20 billion doses are consumed every year around the globe in the form of bio yogurts, fermented dairy drinks, capsules and tablets. According to the World Health Organization, probiotics *by definition* are beneficial for health. Yet the European Food Safety Authority recently refused to accept the evidence for any health claims on product labels. This has caused uproar in academic circles, as swathes of research supported by solid scientific evidence has been rejected and the level of evidence required by the EFSA is widely considered to be too high.

The best evidence comes from a meta-analysis of data from a number of randomized controlled trials, so let's see what these can tell us about the efficacy of probiotics.

Cholesterol A meta-analysis of 13 trials involving 485 participants shows that taking probiotics significantly lowered total cholesterol levels (by 6.4 mg/dl), LDL-cholesterol (by 4.9 mg/dl) and reduced triglycerides by 3.95 mg/dl.

Upper respiratory tract infections A rigorous systematic analysis from the Cochrane Collaboration (an international network of researchers dedicated to providing high-quality evidence to inform healthcare decision making) looked at ten clinical trials involving 3,451 participants. This found that probiotics were better than placebo at reducing the number of episodes of upper respiratory infections such as the common cold. Compared with inactive placebo, taking probiotics daily reduced the risk of having at least one cold by 42 per cent, the risk of having at least three colds by 47 per cent and the chance of needing an antibiotic prescription for an upper respiratory infection by 33 per cent.

Antibiotic-associated diarrhoea Children in hospital receiving broad-spectrum antibiotics can develop diarrhoea as a result of 'killing off' the healthy bacteria in their gut. Co-prescribing probiotics is therefore common in many hospitals worldwide and is a standard part of care in Scandinavia. A meta-analysis of three trials involving 1,092 children showed that those given probiotics for the duration of their hospital stay were 63 per cent less likely to develop diarrhoea and 51 per cent less likely to develop rotavirus gastroenteritis. One in five adults taking antibiotics also develop diarrhoea. A similar meta-analysis of adults showed that co-administration of probiotics reduced the risk by 44 per cent, while for *Clostridium difficile*-associated disease – which can be life-threatening – the relative risk was reduced by 71 per cent. A Cochrane Collaboration systematic review of 63 trials involving 8,014 participants showed that when diarrhoea did occur, probiotics had clear beneficial effects in shortening its duration (by at least 24 hours) and reducing stool frequency with effects noticed by day two. They also noted a lack of side effects and stated that they were safe to use alongside rehydration therapy.

Traveller's diarrhoea A meta-analysis of 12 studies showed that several probiotic bacteria reduced the risk of developing gastro-enteritis when travelling by 15 per cent.

Irritable bowel syndrome A meta-analysis of 14 trials involving over 1,165 people, and another of ten trials involving 918 people showed that probiotics were better than placebo with noticeable improvements in overall symptoms such as pain, flatulence and bloating.

Allergies Mothers-to-be who take probiotics during pregnancy can reduce the chance of their offspring developing allergic conditions such as eczema. This is because, during early development, the immune system has to find a balance between tolerating harmless bacteria while fighting infections, and tolerating harmless dietary and self-identified proteins while attacking foreign proteins. Exposure to beneficial probiotic bacteria appears to help the immune system mature in the correct way. A meta-analysis of seven studies involving 2,843 children whose mothers took probiotics or placebo during pregnancy and breastfeeding showed that taking lactobacilli reduced the risk of developing an allergy by 10.6 per cent.

Prebiotics

Prebiotics are defined as 'non-digestible food ingredients that selectively stimulate a limited number of bacteria in the colon to improve host health'. They are not digested or absorbed, and travel intact to the large bowel where they act as a fermentable food source to stimulate the growth of probiotic bacteria. They cannot be fermented by other, less beneficial bowel bacteria or by potential pathogens, and therefore act as a food to selectively promote the growth of beneficial probiotic bacteria.

Prebiotics include substances known as fructo-oligosaccharides (FOS), which are a form of soluble fibre found in some foods such as oats, barley, wheat, garlic, onions, bananas, honey and tomatoes. Some prebiotics are now being added to breakfast cereals and other 'functional' foods. Probiotics and prebiotics are also increasingly used together, as supplements, in a practice referred to by nutritionists as synbiotics.

Few safety concerns are associated with prebiotics, but it is important that their fermentation should not have undesirable effects on bowel function or habit, or be associated with the production of undesirable products such as excessive gas, which can cause discomfort and bloating. If you choose to take a prebiotic supplement, do not exceed the stated dose.

7

Water, acid, alcohol, salt and additives

Your diet must provide all the ingredients needed for energy and all the processes of life including metabolism, reproduction, growth and repair. So far, we've considered the macronutrients (carbohydrates, proteins, fat, fibre), essential micronutrients (vitamins, minerals) and phytochemicals in the diet. In addition, the diet contributes five other important components: water, acidity, alcohol, salt (at levels well above those needed for essential micronutrient functions) and food additives.

Water

Water is more important for good nutrition than is generally realized. It is essential for energy metabolism in the citric acid cycle, for nutrient transport, waste disposal and the regulation of body temperature through perspiration.

Water contributes 60 per cent of the weight of an average male – a total of 40 to 50 litres – while the weight of the average female is 55 per cent water (33 to 35 litres), due to the relatively greater percentage of body fat.

Two-thirds of your body water is inside your cells, while the remaining third bathes the outside of your cells and flows through your circulation in the so-called 'internal sea' of interstitial fluid. Water molecules constantly move from one fluid compartment to another as nutrients and waste substances are passed to and from your cells.

THE FLUIDS OF LIFE

The body of a man weighing 70 kg contains:

- a total of 42 litres water
- 28 litres within his body cells
- 14 litres outside his body cells, of which 3 to 4 litres are in his circulation

During an averagely active day in a temperate climate the body loses around 2.5 litres of fluid, either through the lungs as water vapour, through the skin as sweat, or through the kidneys as urine. A small amount is also lost through the bowels. If you take vigorous exercise or visit a hot country, it is easy to lose twice this amount. Athletes in hot climates may lose as much as 10 litres of fluid per day.

HOW YOU LOSE WATER

Average daily water losses from the body:

- urine   1,500 ml
- sweat and water vapour from the lungs   800 ml
- in bowel motions   200 ml

Your body normally maintains a fine fluid balance, which is regulated partly by the hormonal control of urine production in the kidneys, and partly by the concentration of salts, sugars and soluble proteins that draw water into your circulation. As long as you replace your daily water losses through adequate drinking and eating, the amount of fluid in your intracellular and extracellular compartments is kept within narrow limits. Excess fluid passes into your circulation and is usually filtered out by the kidneys. If you are dehydrated, you will pass less urine than normal as your body conserves its water stores and triggers a sensation of thirst.

Ideally, men need to obtain at least 2.5 litres of water per day and women 2 litres per day. This is acquired partly from beverages and partly from moisture-rich foods such as soups. Children should drink approximately half this amount, depending on their age. Urine colour is a useful way of checking your hydration status in the workplace – it should be pale in colour. Urine that is dark yellow and concentrated is an important sign of dehydration.

TEA AND HYDRATION

As caffeine has a mild diuretic effect, it is often claimed that caffeinated drinks, such as tea, have a negative effect on hydration. However, research does not support this. A gold-standard randomized, double-blind, placebo-controlled crossover trial involving 21 healthy males aged 20 to 55 years found no difference in hydration levels whether participants drank four mugs (240 ml per mug) of black tea, each containing around 50 mg caffeine, or boiled water (240 ml per mug) at set intervals over one day. Blood samples and a 24-hour urine collection showed no great differences between concentrations of electrolytes, urea, protein or osmolality (a unit of measurement for the amount of a chemical dissolved in a fluid) of body fluids. Urine volume and colour also remained the same. Thus, both tea and water appear to make a similar contribution to fluid requirements that more than offsets the diuretic potential of small caffeine doses.

Although you should ideally drink at least eight glasses of water a day, only one in ten people do so. Over half the population only drink between one and four glasses of water daily.

Unfortunately, thirst receptors are not a sensitive judge of how fluid-deficient you are, and you are already quite dehydrated by the time you feel a craving to drink.

The brain is particularly sensitive to changes in fluid balance. Dehydration is a common cause of tiredness, poor concentration, reduced alertness, reduced short-term memory, headache and mood changes, with increasing agitation, impatience and feelings of stress.

Dehydration also contributes to constipation, kidney stones, and, as it increases the thickness and stickiness of blood, can lead to abnormal blood clotting and even precipitate a heart attack or stroke. Therefore, it is important to drink fluids throughout the day rather than just when you are feeling thirsty.

High ambient temperature can quickly lead to dehydration, so adequate fluid intake is especially important during the summer months or when visiting or living in hot climates. If exposure to heat is excessive, it can lead to heatstroke when increased humidity stops sweat evaporating from the skin to cool the body.

Bottled versus tap water

The purity of drinking water is of paramount importance, and strict directives control the quality of both tap water and bottled water in Europe, the US and other developed countries.

Tap (mains) water is obtained from reservoirs, lakes, rivers and aquifers (which are underground geological formations that store rainwater). Water from these sources is treated to remove harmful substances (e.g. agricultural, industrial or sewage contaminants) and disinfected with chlorine. Tap water is of high quality, but some people dislike the slight smell or taste of chlorine. Placing a covered jug of water in the fridge for around an hour until it is cool will help to remove chlorine traces. Use the cooled water within 24 hours. Using a water filter will also remove chlorine and improve flavour. Table water, offered by some restaurants at a high price, is often just bottled tap water that has been filtered to improve its taste.

FLUORIDATION

In some regions, fluoride is added to public water supplies as fluoridation can help to strengthen teeth, to reduce the risk of dental caries. As another benefit, optimal intakes of fluoride can also strengthen bones and may provide some protection against osteoporotic bone fractures. Excess is harmful, however, and can lead to mottling of developing teeth and, paradoxically, brittleness of bones. Fluoridation is therefore controversial.

Spring water must originate from an underground source and must be microbiologically wholesome in its natural state without the need for any treatments. It may be treated to remove certain minerals or undesirable substances, however. Composition does not have to be specified, and spring water is available as still or sparkling.

SPARKLING OR STILL?

Even naturally sparkling water loses the carbon dioxide gas that provides these bubbles during processing, and this gas must be captured and reintroduced under pressure to produce that delightful effervescence. Carbonated water is more acidic than still water as the carbon dioxide gas dissolves to form weak carbonic acid. This can give a slightly sour taste unless there is sufficient bicarbonate present to reduce the acidity. Check labels for the electrolyte composition of bottled water.

Natural mineral water is bottled at a single, identified and protected source and has a guaranteed consistent composition.

The most important role of water is to act as a solvent for certain mineral salts. When these salts dissolve in water they separate to produce electrically charged particles known as electrolytes. The concentration of different electrolytes in different parts of the body draws water in and out of fluid compartments and maintains the electrical potential across cell membranes, which is vital for life. If fluid or electrolyte levels fall outside narrow limits, metabolic functions are affected in potentially dangerous ways. A low blood calcium level, for example, can cause muscle paralysis, while a high level can cause heart-rhythm abnormalities; a low blood potassium level can cause mental confusion and muscle weakness, while a high blood potassium level can cause the heart to stop beating.

The level of each electrolyte within your cells, the watery part of your blood (serum) and the interstitial fluids bathing your cells is closely regulated in a process known as homeostasis. Homeostatic control mechanisms involve all your internal organs – especially your lungs, liver and kidneys – your endocrine glands and your nervous system.

Blood calcium levels are maintained within a very tight range by calcium-sensing receptors in your parathyroid glands. These trigger the release of parathyroid hormone to increase the amount of calcium released from your bone stores, or calcitonin hormone, which increases the deposition of excess calcium in bones.

Blood water balance is maintained by hormones, which regulate how much urine is lost via your kidneys, and by thirst receptors, which encourage fluid intake. Blood salt levels are regulated by the amount of electrolytes excreted via the kidneys. Hormones such as aldosterone and vasopressin tell the kidneys how much water and electrolytes to reabsorb or excrete. This regulation is closely linked with your blood-pressure control, which is maintained by hormones (renin-angiotensin system) that regulate water and salt balance, by control of your heart rate and through blood-vessel dilation or contraction.

Acidity

Water (H_2O) ionizes into hydrogen ions (H^+, which are also known as protons) and hydroxyl ions (OH^-). It is the concentration of positively charged protons that determines the acidity, or pH, of a fluid. The higher the concentration of protons, the higher the acidity, and vice versa.

The pH scale of a fluid ranges from 0 (highly acid) to 14 (highly alkaline). This is a logarithmic scale, which means that each number represents a tenfold difference in concentration from the numbers on either side. So a liquid with a pH of 5 is 10 times more acidic than a liquid with a pH of 6, and 100 times more acid than a liquid with a pH of 7.

When protons and hydroxyl ions are present in equal proportions, the pH of a fluid is considered neutral with a pH 7 (for example, water). If more H^+ ions are present than OH^- ions, then the fluid is acidic (such as stomach acid). If more OH^- ions than H^+ ions are present, the fluid is alkaline (such as pancreatic secretions).

Many carbonated soft drinks have a pH of 3, making them 10,000 times more acid than water (pH 7). This means they are capable of dissolving tooth enamel and can contribute towards tooth decay.

Dietary acids and enamel

Tooth enamel is the hardest substance found in the body, and forms a thin layer over the surface of each tooth that is up to 2.5 mm thick. Despite its hardness, it readily dissolves on contact with acid substances with a pH of less than 5.5. The acidity of common foods and drinks is surprisingly high. All the substances listed in the chart below have a pH that can harm your teeth with prolonged contact. In fact, someone who eats citrus fruit more than twice a day is 37 times more likely to experience dental erosion than someone who eats citrus fruit less frequently.

Food/drink	pH
Lemon/lime juice	1.8 to 2.4
Fizzy cola drinks	2.7
Orange juice	2.8 to 4.0
Apples	2.9 to 3.5
Grapes	3.3 to 4.5
Mayonnaise	3.8 to 4.0
Tomatoes	3.7 to 4.7
Black coffee	2.4 to 3.3
Vinegar	2.4 to 3.4
Black tea	4.2

Once tooth enamel has dissolved away, it can't be recovered and the softer, underlying parts of the tooth soon start to decay.

Tips to protect your teeth

You don't want to avoid eating fruits and drinking fruit juices altogether, as they form a vital part of a healthy diet. The erosive potential of fruit juices may partly be reduced by diluting them with water, but this may make drinks unacceptable due to their reduced taste and colour. Try to decrease the frequency with which you consume acidic foods or drinks, and consume them quickly, rather than sipping or chewing daintily. Using a straw positioned towards the back of your mouth lessens the contact time between your teeth and the drink compared with using a cup, and may reduce the erosion caused by soft drinks. It also helps to rehydrate your mouth regularly by sipping water. Sluice your mouth out after drinking tea, coffee, cola, sports drinks, wine and other alcoholic drinks. In fact, this is another good reason – apart from responsible drinking – to have a glass of water after each alcoholic drink. You can neutralize acids in your mouth with foods containing calcium and phosphate – some dental experts suggest holding a piece of cheese in your mouth for a few minutes after eating a fruit salad, for example. Another tip is to select fruit juices fortified with added calcium, as this significantly decreases their erosive potential.

You could also brush your teeth with a fluoride toothpaste *before* eating. Don't brush your teeth immediately after eating, as abrasion by a toothbrush after consuming an acidic drink or acidic food may increase loss of enamel. In fact, rinsing your mouth with a glass of water is better than brushing immediately after eating. You could also use a fluoridated mouthwash with a neutral pH.

Floss your teeth regularly to remove the acidic, bacterial plaque that builds up around the teeth. Interdental brushes that clean between your teeth are another new alternative to flossing. As well as reducing gum disease, people who floss regularly appear to be less likely to die from coronary heart disease. As odd as it may seem, this is because having inflamed gums allows mouth bacteria to enter the circulation, where they are believed to trigger arterial disease.

Other health problems associated with an acidic diet

Your body works hard to keep your blood, and the interstitial fluids that bathe your cells, within a very tight pH range of

7.35 to 7.45, which is slightly alkaline. This is achieved by buffering acids with proteins, bicarbonate and other electrolytes such as phosphates; controlling the amount of protons (H^+) and bicarbonate ions (HCO_3^-) eliminated through your kidneys; and regulating the amount of acidic carbon dioxide gas exhaled through your lungs.

Even slight movements outside this narrow blood pH range will severely affect cell function by changing the three-dimensional shapes adopted by important cell proteins and enzymes, and by affecting the electrical balance of nerve and muscle cells.

Your diet strongly influences the amount of acid your body has to process. When a food is broken down, the metabolism of its various building blocks – proteins, carbohydrates and fats – results in either the net production or consumption of protons – the basic unit of acidity. If the metabolism of a food results in the production of excess protons, it is classified as an acid food, although 'acid-forming' is a more accurate description. If the metabolism of a food uses up more protons than it produces, however, then it is classified as an alkaline-forming food.

There is a lot of confusion around the concept of acid and alkaline foods. This is because the acidity of a food refers to its effect on the acidity (pH) of your urine *after* it has been fully processed in your body. Put simply, it's the effect of the 'ash' remaining after that food has been processed to release its energy, micronutrients and salts. It does not refer to whether or not the food itself is acidic or alkaline in quality, nor the effect it has on the acidity of your digestive system or even your blood. In fact, many acid-tasting foods such as lemons, oranges and tomatoes actually have an alkaline effect on the body.

It may seem illogical that acidic-tasting fruits, such as lemons and limes, have an alkaline effect on your urine, but this is easily explained. The types of acid present in fruits, such as citric acid and malic acid, are weak acids. This means they do not separate out into their ions to release protons (H^+) to any great extent. Instead, they are readily neutralized by the large amount of potassium and sodium also present in the fruit to form salts such as potassium citrate and potassium malate. During metabolism, these salts react with sodium, water and carbon dioxide in your cells to form sodium bicarbonate, which has an alkaline effect on urine. Adding sugar to fruit juices reduces the buffering effect of potassium, however, so sweetened fruit juices become acid-forming.

Protein-rich foods such as meat and dairy products are the main acid-forming foods in your diet. This is because the amino acids they contain are broken down to produce excess protons, which your body excretes via your urine. These are therefore classed as 'acid' or 'acid-forming' foods. When healthy, your liver, kidneys and lungs can process acid-forming foods without undue difficulty.

Having to process excess acid-forming foods can lead to some loss of bone-mineral density when phosphate salts are leached out to buffer excess acids in the body. Phosphate is stored in your bones and teeth as calcium phosphate, so when phosphate is used to buffer acid-forming foods, calcium is left behind which, in some cases, may contribute to the formation of kidney stones. Eating an acid-forming diet may also increase the level of inflammation in the body, thus increasing the risk of a number of health conditions.

A growing body of research now suggests that the long-term consumption of an acid-forming diet may have other adverse effects on health. This becomes more of a problem as you get older, when your kidney function naturally declines and becomes less able to secrete the excess acid from your body.

Acid diet and osteoporosis

There is growing evidence that an acid-forming diet is harmful for bones. The average Western diet supplies notable quantities of acid (50 to 100 milliequivalents acid per day), which contributes to a low-grade, long-term metabolic acidosis. Because bone is used to buffer this excess acid, it leads to gradual dissolution of bone mineral and reduced bone mass. In healthy male volunteers, for example, eating an acid-forming diet increased their urinary calcium excretion by 74 per cent compared to when they consumed an alkaline-forming diet. This extra calcium was essentially leached from their bones. Studies in which bone density has been measured by ultrasound or dual-energy X-ray absorptiometry has also shown a correlation between the nutritional acid load and bone health. To help protect your bones, aim to consume less acid-forming foods (protein-rich foods) and more alkaline-forming foods such as fruit and vegetables, which are associated with a more alkaline environment and have been shown to have a beneficial effect on bone health. In addition, drinking an alkaline, bicarbonate-rich water has also been shown to have a beneficial effect on reducing bone loss and, in those with an acid-forming diet, mineral-water consumption has been suggested as an easy and inexpensive way of helping to prevent osteoporosis.

Acid diet and liver health

Excess intakes of acid-forming foods have been associated with a build-up of fat in the liver, which is involved in processing proteins from which the acidic protons are released. In adolescents, females with the most acid-forming diets are 4.5 times more likely to show liver enzyme changes associated with non-alcoholic fatty liver disease than those with the least acid diet. Further studies are needed to confirm these findings.

Acid diet and heart disease

Mild metabolic acidosis is associated with a number of heart-disease risk factors – possibly because it increases your secretion of the stress hormone, cortisol. A recent study published in the *British Journal of Nutrition* involving 1,136 female dietetic students in Japan found that acid-forming diets were associated with a higher blood pressure, total and LDL-cholesterol, body mass index (BMI) and waist circumference – even after adjusting for other confounding variables such as smoking and physical activity level. Although this is an observational study and no definite links can be drawn, it adds to the body of evidence that a more alkaline-forming diet is most beneficial for health.

Acid diet and Alzheimer's disease

An acid-forming diet affects the way metal ions are handled in the body, and is associated with higher blood and brain concentrations of aluminium than an alkaline-forming diet. This has been suggested as one cause of the neurological damage associated with Alzheimer's disease. Although it is by no means proven, it is another potential reason to start thinking about eating less acid-forming foods and more alkaline-forming foods.

Some nutritionists and naturopathic doctors suggest following a diet that consists of 60 to 80 per cent alkaline foods and only 20 to 40 per cent acid foods. This is controversial among 'orthodox' nutritionists and doctors, who are unaware of the growing evidence for harm due to chronic, low-grade metabolic acidosis in the body. But, as it basically means eating more fruit and green leafy vegetables and cutting back on the amount of animal proteins and processed foods you eat, this approach to nutrition is exactly the one that orthodox clinicians suggest, although they may not be aware of all the mechanisms underpinning the benefits of those five portions a day.

The main dietary sources of acids and alkalis are shown in Table 11.

Table 11 Acid-forming and alkaline-forming foods

Strongly acid-forming foods
Animal proteins (eggs, poultry, meats, seafood); beer; coffee; sugar; sweetened fruit juice; black tea; highly processed foods, carbonated soft drinks such as colas; artificial sweeteners; white vinegar; sauerkraut

Mildly acid-forming foods
Grains (barley, oats, quinoa, rice, wheat, flours, bread, pasta); some pulses (black beans, chickpeas, kidney beans); most nuts (pecans, cashews, peanuts, pistachios, walnuts); most dairy products (cream, cheese, milk, ice-cream, yogurt); wine; apple cider vinegar; sparkling water; vegetable oils

Neutral
Distilled water

Mildly alkaline-forming foods
Green tea; tomatoes; low-sugar fruits; berries; citrus fruit; figs; peppers; some pulses (alfalfa, lentils, lima beans, soybeans, navy beans); tofu; some nuts (almonds, pine nuts, chestnuts, coconut); onions; turnip; swede; potatoes and other root vegetables; cabbage, bicarbonate-rich mineral water

Strongly alkaline-forming foods
Green leafy vegetables (kale, broccoli, spinach, barley grass, wheat grass); herbs (parsley, coriander leaf, oregano); avocados; celery; asparagus; green beans; beetroot; radishes; garlic

Alcohol

Interest in the potential health benefits of alcohol initially arose because of the so-called French Paradox. Compared with Britain and the US, the French eat as much saturated fat, have similar high cholesterol levels, smoke as much (if not more), take as little exercise and drink significantly more wine, yet their risk of coronary heart disease is lower. In fact, Le Paradoxe Français was most evident in Gascony – home of the fatty saucisses de Toulouse and the cardiologist's ultimate nightmare, pâté de foie gras. Researchers concluded that the most obvious explanation for this French paradox was red wine consumption. More recent data suggests that any form of alcohol, whether beer, wine or spirits, can prove beneficial – but only when consumed in moderation.

A large 2008 meta-analysis that pooled data from 34 studies involving over a million people, found that the risk of coronary heart disease decreased with intakes of up to four drinks per day in men and two drinks per day in women. Higher intakes were associated with increased mortality related to abnormal heart rhythms, high blood pressure, liver disease and, in women, an increased risk of breast cancer. A more recent 2011 meta-analysis published in the *British Medical Journal* confirmed that, compared with teetotallers, people with a light to moderate alcohol intake appear to have a 29 per cent lower chance of developing coronary heart disease and a 25 per cent reduced risk of dying from it. The lowest risk for heart disease occurred with one to two drinks per day, but for stroke mortality the lowest risk was for those who drank around one drink per day.

Alcohol also appears to have beneficial effects on factors associated with hardening and furring-up of the arteries (atherosclerosis), raising levels of 'good' HDL-cholesterol, lowering levels of a blood-clotting factor called fibrinogen and discouraging arterial calcification.

Overall, evidence suggests that moderate drinking (one to two units per day) is especially beneficial for men over 40 years of age and post-menopausal women. However, recent research suggests that the benefits of moderate alcohol intake do not apply equally to all people. In fact, those most likely to benefit are those who follow an unhealthy diet and lifestyle, who take little exercise or who smoke. Little additional benefit from alcohol is seen in those who do not smoke, eat fruit and vegetables daily and who exercise for three or more hours per week, probably because they are already obtaining the maximum benefits possible from following a healthy lifestyle.

Drinking excess alcohol can deplete the body of vitamin C and vitamins from the B group, which are used in its metabolism. Alcohol can also contribute to gaining weight and obesity. As an energy source, alcohol provides 7 kcal (29.4 kJ) per gram – more than protein and carbohydrate, but less than fat.

KNOW YOUR UNITS

In the UK, a unit of alcohol is equivalent to 10 ml or 8 g of pure alcohol. Half a pint (300 ml) of beer, lager or cider that is 3.5 per cent alcohol in strength contains one unit. But many lagers now contain 5 per cent alcohol, and some versions supply as much as 9 per cent alcohol. One small (100 ml) glass of wine that is 10 per cent alcohol in strength contains one unit. But most wines are now much stronger (12 per cent to 15 per cent alcohol) and many pubs sell wine in 250 ml glasses. Depending on its percentage alcohol content, a bottle of wine typically contains between 8 and 11 units of alcohol. A 25 ml bar or pub measure of 40 per cent spirit contains one unit. But many bars and pubs now serve 35 ml measures as standard, and will often serve a double unless you specifically say you want a single. To calculate how much you are drinking, use the handy unit calculator at www.drinkaware.co.uk.

NB In the US the term 'drink' is used as a unit of alcohol, and usually means 14 g of alcohol, while in Australia a unit is 10 g.

Salt

Common table salt – known chemically as sodium chloride – is added to processed food to enhance flavour, act as a stabilizer, retain moisture and help products last longer on the shelf. It is also used to preserve foods such as fish and meats, as bacteria and moulds that would spoil these foods cannot grow in very salty environments. In fact, salt was so highly valued in fridge-free

Ancient Rome, that soldiers received a salt allowance as part of their pay. They were literally 'worth their salt'.

In the body, salt dissolves to form two electrolytes, sodium (Na^+) and chloride (Cl^-). Most sodium in the body is found outside your cells in the interstitial fluids and blood. Very little sodium is present inside your cells as millions of tiny salt pumps in cell membranes force sodium out of your cells in exchange for potassium ions. This action means the inside of every cell develops a small, negative electric charge, which is vital for life. Without it, your nerve and brain cells couldn't pass messages to one another, and heart muscle cells would not be able to contract. Common salt is therefore essential for good health. So much so that the transport of salt in and out of our cells is one of the main energy-consuming processes in our body. It is estimated to account for 33 per cent of our daily energy needs.

Before the advent of processed and fast food, we obtained our salt from adding it to preserve foods, during cooking and at the table. Now these sources are minimal compared to the amount of salt consumed in processed foods. For example, a typical microwave meal contains around 5 g salt, a bowl of breakfast cereal provides 1 g while a serving of canned soup gives 2 g.

Humans evolved on a diet providing less than 1 g salt per day. The average Western diet currently provides as much as 10 g salt per day or more. This tenfold rise in sodium intake is responsible for the age-related rise in blood pressure seen in Western populations, as the kidneys of many people are unable to excrete the additional salt load. The retained salt stimulates thirst and promotes fluid retention, which causes blood pressure to rise.

Populations with salt intakes of less than 3 g per day do not show increased blood presure with increasing age. Yanomamo Indians, for example, whose traditional diet contains less than 1 g of salt per day have an average blood pressure of 96/60 mmHg and do not develop hypertension. Populations following a Western-style diet that is high in salt typically have a blood pressure of around 140/90 mmHg, which is the borderline above which a diagnosis of high blood pressure (hypertension) is made if the high readings are consistent.

Not adding salt during cooking, or at the table, can lower systolic blood pressure (the peak pressure achieved as your heart beats) by as much as 5 mmHg. If everyone did this, it is estimated that the incidence of stroke in the population would be reduced by as much as 26 per cent and coronary heart disease by 15 per cent. Since eight times more dietary salt is present in processed foods, the effects of cutting back on these is even greater.

Research suggests that a realistic sodium reduction (equivalent to cutting out 4.6 g salt per day) over at least four weeks can lower blood pressure by an average of 2.03/0.97 mmHg for those with normal blood pressures, and by 4.96/2.73 mmHg in those with hypertension. Reducing salt intake by 6 g salt per day was predicted to lower blood pressure by 3.57/1.66 mmHg for people with normal blood pressure, and by 7.11/3.88 mmHg in those with hypertension.

Salt restriction can reduce the dose and number of drugs needed to control high blood pressure. Recent research also indicates that people whose high blood pressure does not respond to multiple medications are likely to be eating too much salt, which suggests that the fluid retention associated with a high dietary salt intake is counteracting the effects of medication. This is supported by the fact that sodium restriction can produce sharp reductions in blood pressure in these cases of up to 22.7/9.1 mmHg.

Dietary salt intake is also strongly correlated with the thickness of the wall of the left ventricle of the heart (which has to pump a larger volume of blood out into the body) and, in people with hypertension, a high sodium intake is associated with a decreased diameter and increased stiffness of the arteries, whether or not atherosclerosis is present.

Overall, it is estimated that reducing your salt intake by 3 g per day (for example, from 12 g down to 9 g) would reduce your risk of a stroke by 13 per cent, and your risk of a heart attack by 10 per cent. Restricting salt intake down to 6 g per day could double this preventive effect, while restricting salt intake to 3 g daily might triple the benefits.

EXCESS DIETARY SALT

A high intake of salt has also been linked with other health problems such as bone-thinning (osteoporosis, as sodium increases calcium losses through the kidney), fluid retention (equivalent to 1 kg to 2 kg at some times of the month for women), asthma, congestive heart failure, liver cirrhosis and even stomach cancer.

How much salt do you need?

An average male weighing 70 kg has around 225 g salt in his body, and can maintain a healthy sodium balance with an intake of as little as 1.25 g salt per day – as long as he does not sweat heavily. Ideally, an adult should obtain no more than 6 g salt per day – around one level teaspoon. Target maximum intakes for children are proportionately smaller, as shown in Table 12.

Table 12 Suggested maximum salt intakes according to age

Age	Target salt intake (grams per day)
0 to 6 months	less than 1 g daily
7 to 12 months	1 g per day
1 to 3 years	2 g per day
4 to 6 years	3 g daily
7 to 10 years	5 g daily
Over 11 years	6 g daily (as per adults)

Most dietary salt (around 75 per cent) is hidden in processed foods including canned products, ready-prepared meals, biscuits, cakes and breakfast cereals. Some foods are 30 per cent more salty than seawater, which provides 2.5 g salt per 100 g water. Checking labels of bought products and avoiding those containing high amounts of salt is vital to influence your salt intake. A good general rule is that, per 100 g food (or per serving if a serving is less than 100 g):

- 0.5 g sodium (1.25 g salt) or more is a lot of sodium
- 0.1 g sodium (0.25 g salt) or less is a little sodium

To convert 'sodium' to salt content, simply multiply by 2.5, so that, for example, a serving of soup containing 0.4 g sodium actually provides 1 g salt (sodium chloride).

Salt is easily replaceable with herbs and spices such as black pepper. When cutting back on salt, it takes around a month to retrain your taste buds, and food may taste bland initially until your taste buds start responding to lower salt concentrations. Try adding lime juice to food, which stimulates tastes buds and decreases the amount of salt you need, too.

The importance of potassium

Where salt is essential, use mineral-rich rock salt rather than table salt, or use a low-sodium, higher-potassium brand of salt sparingly. Potassium helps to flush excess sodium from the body via the kidneys, and a diet that is lacking in potassium is linked with a higher risk of high blood pressure and stroke, especially if your diet is also high in sodium. In one study, people taking medication for high blood pressure were able to reduce their drug dose by half – under medical supervision – after increasing the potassium content of their food. Good sources of potassium include seafood, fresh fruit, vegetables, juices and wholegrains.

To cut back on salt intake avoid:

- adding salt during cooking or at the table
- obviously salty foods such as crisps, bacon, salted nuts
- tinned products, especially those canned in brine
- cured, smoked or pickled fish and meats
- meat pastes, pâtés
- ready-prepared meals
- packet soups and sauces
- stock cubes and yeast extracts
- check all labels and select brands with the lowest salt content

Other food additives

As well as adding salt to processed foods, manufacturers also add a variety of different chemicals to enhance colour and flavour and to preserve products for a longer shelf life. These additives are displayed on labels with identification codes based on an international numbering system. In the European Union, the numbers are prefixed with the letter E, but in the US the number alone is used. Some additives are natural, but many are artificial and would not otherwise feature in the diet. The number classifications are available on the internet:

Europe
http://www.food.gov.uk/policy-advice/additivesbranch/
    enumberlist#.UKeOpYawRMc

United States
http://www.fda.gov/food/foodingredientspackaging/ucm
    115326.htm

Australia
http://www.foodstandards.gov.au/consumerinformation/
    additives/

Food additives are generally recognized as safe. However, they have been linked with health problems in some people. Research looking at the effects of artificial food additives in the diet of almost 2,000 young children, for example, found that eliminating artificial colourings and benzoate preservatives produced significant improvements in behaviour, with less hyperactivity.

Monosodium glutamate (MSG) is an amino–acid flavour enhancer used in Asian cuisine. It stimulates specific taste-bud receptors to induce a savoury or meaty taste known in Japan as *umami*. Consuming MSG increases blood levels of the amino acid, glutamate. This acts as a building block for making the neurotransmitter acetylcholine which, in some people, can cause headache and may trigger asthma in those sensitive to its effects. Studies are inconclusive, however, and it has been suggested that this sensitivity may only occur in those with a deficiency of vitamin B6, or after consuming MSG on an empty stomach, or with alcohol, which hastens its absorption.

MONOSODIUM GLUTAMATE

MSG may appear on food labels as monosodium glutamate, sodium glutamate, 2-aminoglutaric acid or as additive number E621. It is also present in flavourings described as: hydrolyzed vegetable protein (HVP), hydrolyzed plant protein (HPP) and 'Natural Flavour'. People who are highly sensitive to MSG may also react to other glutamic acid salts. The names and E numbers to look for are:

E620 glutamic acid
E621 monosodium glutamate
E622 monopotassium glutamate
E624 monoammonium glutamate
E625 magnesium diglutamate

Some people with asthma are sensitive to benzoates, especially if they are also sensitive to aspirin. Benzoates are among the most commonly used food additives. These preservatives are used to prevent the growth of bacteria, yeasts and fungi in many foods and drinks, especially those that are acidic. Benzoyl peroxide is also used as a bleaching agent in flours, breads and some cheeses such as soft Italian cheeses, blue cheeses (especially Gorgonzola) and feta cheese. The way in which benzoates can trigger asthma is unknown, but may involve the production of inflammatory chemicals.

BENZOATES

These may appear on labels as any of the following:

E210 benzoic acid
E211 sodium benzoate
E212 potassium benzoate
E213 calcium benzoate
E214 ethyl paraben (ethyl para-hydroxybenzoate)
E215 sodium ethyl para-hydroxybenzoate
E216 propylparaben (propyl para-hydroxybenzoate)
E217 sodium propyl para-hydroxybenzoate
E218 methyl paraben (methyl para-hydroxybenzoate)
E219 sodium methyl para-hydroxybenzoate

In addition, as many as one in ten people with asthma are sensitive to sulphites, especially those whose asthma requires steroid treatments or who are sensitive to aspirin. Sulphites (or sulfites) are antioxidant preservatives used to preserve colour, slow the browning of fruit, vegetables and seafood, and to bleach food starches and bread dough. At one time, they were widely added to fresh fruit and vegetables, especially lettuce. As a result of an increase in sensitivity reactions, however, their use was restricted during the mid-1980s and they are now only used where no suitable alternative exists.

When sulphites dissolve in the mouth during chewing, sulphuric acid is formed, which releases sulphur dioxide gas. When inhaled, this noxious gas irritates hypersensitive airways to cause spasm. Sulphites also interact with proteins on cell membranes, and may alter them sufficiently to be seen as 'foreign' and trigger an allergic reaction. Another theory is that some people with asthma only produce low levels of an enzyme (sulphite oxidase) which is needed to convert sulphites to inert sulphates.

SULPHITING AGENTS

Sulphiting agents that are used in the food and drinks industry may be shown on labels as follows:

E220 sulphur dioxide
E221 sodium sulphite
E222 sodium bisulphite (sodium hydrogen sulphite)
E223 sodium metabisulphite
E224 potassium metabisulphite
E225 potassium sulphite
E226 calcium sulphite
E227 calcium hydrogen sulphite
E228 potassium hydrogen sulphite

Sulphur and sulphites may be spelled as sulfur or sulfites on labels.

NB Sulphates (sulfates) are *not* associated with sensitivity reactions.

Organic foods

According to the Soil Association, the UK's leading charity campaigning for healthy, sustainable food, record numbers of people are now choosing to eat a wholesome, natural, organic diet because they feel that by doing this they are making a healthier choice.

What does 'organic' mean?

Organic foods are produced using sustainable farming practices without the use of agricultural chemicals (pesticides, weedkillers, fungicides, fumigants, antibiotics, hormonal growth promoters, artificial fertilizers), genetic manipulation, irradiation or undue exposure to environmental pollution. In their place, farmers use traditional methods of pest control, crop rotation, rotation with green-manure crops such as clover (which fix nitrogen in the soil and thereby act as natural fertilizers), careful timing of sowing and allowing land to lie fallow. This results in products that are full of flavour, in comparison to their non-organic counterparts, vitamins and minerals and which contain the lowest possible amounts of artificial chemicals.

In contrast, non-organically grown produce is regularly treated from the time the crop is in seed form, during germination and throughout its growing cycle. A non-organic apple, for example, is typically dosed around 40 times with up to 100 additives before you eat it. These chemicals do not just lie on the surface of the produce, but are found beneath the skin and sometimes throughout the flesh itself. A typical non-organic lettuce is sprayed with artificial fertilizers and pesticides an average of 11 times in the few weeks it takes to develop, while a Cox's apple is sprayed 16 times with 36 different active pesticide ingredients before you pick it up and eat it. And apples on the outside of the tree can receive 13 times the amount of spray present on those near the inside of the tree. These treatments are designed to boost growth and prevent attack from moulds and insects. In contrast, organic crops are either not sprayed at all, or are treated with a tightly regulated list of organic products such as pyrethrum (a Chrysanthemum extract), neem oil (from neem-tree seeds) or beneficial soil bacteria (e.g. *Bacillus thuringiensis*) that kill weevils without harming humans.

The full effects of many chemicals on long-term health are still not fully understood. Some researchers suggest that 60 per cent of all herbicides, 90 per cent of all fungicides and 30 per cent of all insecticides can potentially cause cancer, but the mutagenicity of most pesticides is unknown because it has not been studied. Consuming more than one toxin at the same time may magnify their toxic effects.

Limits on the level of pesticide and herbicide residues in food are set for health reasons, but these assume that chemicals are properly used. If improperly used, serious harm may result. You might assume that improper use is rare, but unfortunately this is not the case. Testing of non-organic fruit and vegetables on sale in the UK has found that nearly half (48 per cent) contained detectable pesticide residues, as did over a quarter (28.6 per cent) of other foods tested, including cereals, meat, dairy, fish and processed foods. Many samples of lettuce, apples, oranges and pears contained residues of between three and seven different pesticides. Although each individual chemical was present at safe levels, American researchers have found that combining pesticides at safe levels can multiply their toxicity and may have effects on reproductive- , immune- and nervous-system function. Concern was sufficient for the UK government to recommend washing and peeling fruit before eating 'as a sensible precaution' – especially when preparing them for children – and that topping and tailing carrots was also a good idea to reduce exposure to residues, although the advice was subsequently withdrawn as many nutrients are stored just beneath the skin, and peeling will not remove residues that have a 'systemic' effect, which means that they are designed to be taken up into the plant and therefore found not just on the surface, but throughout their entire flesh. Unfortunately, washing with water alone does not remove residues altogether as those used have been formulated to resist being washed off by rain. According to the Soil Association, after washing with water between 50 and 93 per cent of residues remain on potatoes, apples and broccoli. Blanching in hot water and cooking can remove significant amounts of some pesticide residues, however.

Although the adverse health effects of agricultural residues in the diet are not known, a number of researchers have linked them with symptoms such as headache, tremor, lack of energy, muscle weakness, depression, anxiety, poor memory, nausea and diarrhoea, plus reduced male fertility, suppressed immunity and cancer. Much of this evidence comes from environmental and occupational exposure studies in agricultural workers. Whether dietary exposure from residues on foods can cause similar effects is less easy to confirm as data is incomplete.

HOW MUCH IS TOO MUCH?

It's estimated that, during the course of one year, those following a non-organic diet consume around 6 kg of chemicals such as food additives, colourings, flavourings, preservatives, waxes, fertilizers, pesticides and herbicide residues.

Nutritional quality of organic versus non-organic foods

Evidence from over 400 published papers suggests that there are notable nutritional differences between organic and non-organic foods. Although some academics argue that these are confounded by differences in water content (organic produce tends to contain less water and is therefore more nutrient-dense) this still means that, per serving, you are obtaining less water and more nutrients. In addition, at least 22 studies have compared the vitamin and mineral content of organic and non-organic fruit and vegetables using dry matter only, and eight have similarly compared the vitamin, mineral and protein content of cereals. Having taken water out of the equation, these consistently suggest that organic produce contains more minerals (especially phosphorus, potassium, calcium, magnesium, zinc) and more vitamin C. In one study, organic cherry tomatoes, for example, contained 4.5 per cent more potassium, 129 per cent more calcium and 65 per cent more zinc than in those grown traditionally, although the manganese content was 11 per cent lower.

Several studies also suggest that organically grown fruit and vegetables contain higher amounts of phytochemicals such as carotenoids (e.g. betacarotene, lycopene) and phenols. This is not surprising, given that plants not dosed with synthetic pesticides are likely to need to produce more of their own natural antioxidant defences.

To limit your exposure to dietary agrochemicals, you may want to consider buying organically grown versions when you can. Although organic produce can be more expensive, you can keep your costs down if you buy fruit and vegetables in season rather than those imported at additional cost; buy locally; buy in bulk; buy wholefoods rather than processed foods; eat more plant-based foods and less meat; look out for special offers; join a box scheme that delivers fruit and vegetables to your door from local producers.

8

What is a balanced diet?

The human body evolved on a diet that was high in lean protein derived from animals, game birds and fish. The diet followed by Stone Age hunter-gatherers provided relatively few carbohydrates, most of which came from green leafy vegetables such as purslane (also rich in vitamins C and E – a succulent leaf resembling a fleshy lamb's lettuce, currently considered a weed in most of the world but still eaten around the Mediterranean and in parts of Asia and Mexico), berries and a few low-glycaemic wild grains, with very little in the way of sugar and refined carbohydrates such as those we eat today. And the fats within the Palaeolithic diet were mostly polyunsaturated omega-3s plus monounsaturates, with far fewer of the omega-6s and saturated fats that we consume now. With the agricultural revolution 10,000 years ago, we started eating more wholegrains and cultivated crops, and becoming less active as humans settled down into subsistence-farming communities. Following the industrial revolution, processing of grains became common and more and more of the fibre- and mineral-rich husks we used to eat were discarded. Within the space of 500 generations, our diet and lifestyle has changed enormously, but the human genome has stayed relatively unchanged. At the same time, modern humans are more than 60 per cent more sedentary than our hunter-gatherer ancestors, but we are still programmed to engage in a greater degree of physical exercise. This mismatch between our current diet and lifestyle and our Palaeolithic genes has been blamed for a multitude of modern health issues such as obesity, high blood pressure, diabetes and coronary heart disease. Many nutritionists, therefore, urge us to return to our roots with a more balanced wholefood diet that more closely resembles the one enjoyed by our great-great ancestors.

Achieving balance

Every cell in your body today – even those in your skeleton – is made up of different molecules to those that were present a year ago. Even the inert parts of your skeleton – the calcium-containing mineral, hydroxyapatite – is turned over slowly at a rate of 10 per cent annually, meaning that every ten years your entire bone-mineral stores are replaced. All these new building blocks ultimately come from your diet. So your food needs to provide all the energy, essential fatty acids, essential amino acids, vitamins and minerals you need for optimum health.

A nutritionally balanced diet is one that provides everything you need, without containing too much or too little of any component. It will contain sufficient

- energy (from carbohydrates, proteins and fats) to fuel your basal metabolic rate, level of physical activity and maintain a healthy weight
- protein (especially the essential amino acids) for tissue repair, regeneration and rejuvenation
- fat (especially the essential fatty acids) for hormone balance and healthy cell membranes throughout the body, including the brain and retina
- vitamins and minerals to meet your daily requirement
- phytochemicals, especially the antioxidants, for immune health
- fibre and probiotics for digestive health
- water, protons and electrolytes to maintain normal hydration, body fluid and acid balance.

Different people require different amounts of each individual nutrient depending on their level of physical activity – both at work and in leisure – their height, weight, age and the genes they have inherited. Healthy-eating guidelines have to meet the needs of all members of the population, and this is not an easy task.

Healthy-eating guidelines

A number of organizations around the world have published healthy-eating guidelines in an attempt to define the optimum healthy diet. These vary in complexity from broad statements aimed at guiding your general choice of food (e.g. eat as wide a variety of foods as possible), to more complex statements that refer to recommended percentage energy intakes from different food groups (e.g. saturated fats should make up no more than 10 per cent of your daily calories). The problem is that neither of these approaches results in a practical understanding of how to eat better. The former is too simplistic to take seriously, and the latter too complex to be clearly understood by most people.

In the UK, the Department of Health launched the Eatwell Plate in 2007 as a visual guide to the relative amounts of each food group your diet should contain (see Diagram 9).

The Eatwell Plate shows how much of what you eat should come from each food group. This includes everything you eat during the day, including snacks, and is much easier to understand at a glance. This tool is far more useful in helping people to select a nutritionally balanced diet, as it encourages you to eat the correct proportion of fruit and vegetables; starchy foods such as bread, rice, potatoes and pasta, with an emphasis on choosing wholegrain varieties whenever you can; milk and dairy foods; meat, fish, eggs, beans and other non-dairy sources of protein; along with just a small amount of foods and drinks that are high in fat and/or sugar.

The eatwell plate

Use the eatwell plate to help you get the balance right. It shows how much of what you eat should come from each food group.

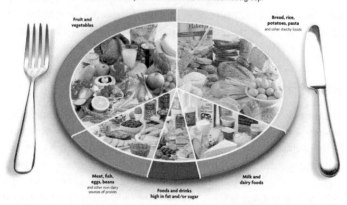

Diagram 9 The UK Eatwell Plate
© Crown copyright. Department of Health in association with the Welsh Assembly Government, the Scottish Government and the Food Standards Agency in Northern Ireland.

Another popular depiction of a healthy diet is the food pyramid, adopted in the US in 1992. In the original, the base of the pyramid consisted of starchy carbohydrates (brown rice, wholemeal bread, wholewheat pasta, wholegrain cereals) with a suggestion to eat six to eleven servings per day. Next up is the fruit and vegetable group, with a suggestion to eat three to five servings of vegetables and two to four of fruit per day. Above this are the animal and dairy products, of which it is recommended that you limit these to two to three servings of milk, yogurt and cheese, plus two to three servings of meat, poultry, fish, pulses, eggs and nuts per day. Finally, the apex of the pyramid contains fats, oils, sugars and sweets, which should be used and consumed sparingly (see Diagram 10).

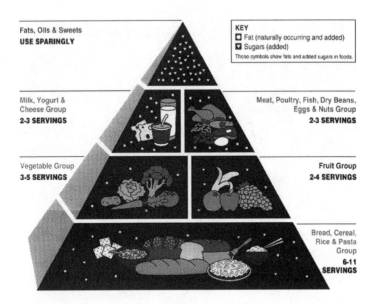

Diagram 10 Original US food pyramid
© U.S. Department of Agriculture. MyPyramid.gov website. Washington, DC.

However, this approach was criticized as it does not differentiate between potentially harmful fats such as trans fats and excess saturated fats, and the beneficial monounsaturated fats such as olive oil or omega-3 fish oils. There is also a lack of clarity as the two to three servings of protein-rich foods was intended as a maximum and the two to four portions of fruit as a minimum. As a result, the Food Pyramid was replaced in 2005 by a more personalized version known as MyPyramid (see Diagram 11) which also stresses the importance of physical activity.

An accompanying website, www.mypyramid.gov, provided detailed information about the different food groups and the daily recommended intake for different ages and genders. For example, women aged 19 to 50 years should obtain 6 oz equivalents

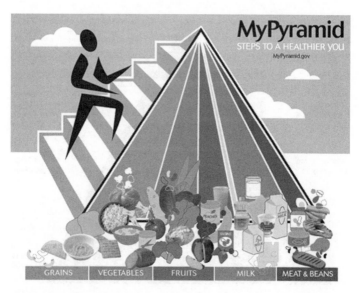

Diagram 11 MyPyramid
© U.S. Department of Agriculture. MyPyramid.gov website. Washington, DC. www.mypyramid.gov (accessed 22 March 2011).

of grains per day, while men aged 19 to 30 years should aim for 8 oz equivalents, and those aged 31 to 50 should obtain 7 oz equivalents (where 1 oz equivalent is 1 slice of bread, 1 cup of ready-to-eat cereal, ½ cup cooked rice, cooked pasta or cooked cereal), of which at least half should be wholegrain products.

Despite being more accurate, this approach was seen by many as unduly complicated. Individuals had to obtain a personalized eating plan by inputting data via the website such as their age, weight, height, gender, level of physical activity and whether or not they wanted to lose some weight. As a result, US nutrition guidelines have now come full circle and returned to a simplistic approach with the introduction of MyPlate, which replaced MyPyramid in June 2011. MyPlate essentially shows a plate divided into four sections, helping people to select a diet that provides around 30 per cent grains, 30 per cent vegetables, 20 per cent fruit and 20 per cent protein. A small additional circle represents dairy intake, such as a glass of low-fat milk or a serving of yogurt. How to use MyPlate is fully explained at www.choosemyplate.gov.

Why select 'brown' wholegrains rather than 'white' processed grains?

Wholegrains form the foundation of a healthy diet as they supply energy in the form of starchy carbohydrates, small amounts of protein and healthy fats (mostly monounsaturated, polyunsaturated fatty acids) plus vitamins, minerals, trace elements and fibre. In fact, brown or wholemeal versions of rice, pasta and bread supply twice as much fibre, and have a lower glycaemic load than their more processed 'white' counterparts, whose fibre- and mineral-rich husks are stripped out during processing.

Rice is a staple food for over half the world's population, for whom it provides both energy and an important source of protein. But its nutritional value is greatly reduced when it is milled to remove the bran, which provides fibre, B-group vitamins and minerals such as calcium, zinc and magnesium. The B-group vitamins are locked into the bran and are only released into the grain when cooked. As a result, those who eat white rice may be at risk of the vitamin-B deficiency disease beriberi, while those who eat brown rice, or rice that was parboiled before milling, are not. Parboiled rice is usually referred to as 'easy cook' rice.

As a result of the industrial revolution, milling boosted the glycaemic index of dietary carbohydrate leading to an estimated threefold increase in the rise of blood glucose levels after a meal (postprandial glycaemia) and insulin secretion. With the advent of fast foods, confectionery and supersized meals, the glycaemic index of the typical Western diet increased even further, leading to widespread 'epidemics' of obesity, glucose intolerance, insulin resistance and Type 2 diabetes.

Until as recently as 2004, healthy-eating recommendations suggested eating at least 55 per cent of calories as carbohydrate, emphasizing the quantity rather than the quality of carbohydrate consumed. It is only since 2005 that recommendations have started to focus on the type of carbohydrate consumed, and suggested that use of glycaemic index/glycaemic load would be more beneficial for health than considering total carbohydrates alone. Much of this change resulted from the popularity of low-carbohydrate diets, such as Atkins, which attracted a negative academic response and prompted a flurry of nutritional studies. Contrary to the entrenched carbohydrate-based paradigm, these started to show that a diet that supplied less than the usually recommended 45 per cent to 65 per cent energy from carbohydrates was associated with improved glucose control and triglyceride levels, 'good' HDL-cholesterol levels and could help some people lose weight. These studies also helped to underpin the growing recognition that a diet providing excess carbohydrates may have contributed towards the rise in obesity, Type 2 diabetes and non-alcoholic fatty liver disease.

We are now moving towards dietary recommendations that are based on quality rather than quantity of macronutrients as wholegrain cereals, unsaturated (i.e. polyunsaturated or mono-unsaturated) fat and protein play a beneficial role in promoting weight loss, insulin sensitivity, glucose tolerance and improved heart-disease risk factors such as lower blood pressure, cholesterol levels, inflammation and incidence of Type 2 diabetes.

Wholegrains and glucose control

Due to the fibre content and lower glycaemic load, the 'brown' wholemeal versions of grain-based foods fill you up for longer and have less impact on blood glucose levels so that less insulin is secreted, less glucose is pushed into adipose (fat) cells and appetite is suppressed for longer. As a result, a diet based on wholegrain products is associated with fewer long-term health problems such as obesity and Type 2 diabetes. This is why they are now seen as the foundation stone of a healthy but varied diet.

In 2004, a study published by the American Diabetes Association looked at 36,787 men and women without diabetes and followed them for four years. Those with the highest intake of white bread were 37 per cent more likely to develop diabetes over this period than those with the lowest intake. The researchers concluded that lowering the glycaemic index of the diet could reduce the risk of Type 2 diabetes, even when a high carbohydrate intake was maintained, and that one way to achieve this would be to substitute white bread for breads with a lower GI value.

Wholegrains and cardiovascular disease

Researchers now know that a high-glycaemic diet promotes obesity, insulin resistance, increases the production of triglyceride fats and small, dense LDL-cholesterol particles in the liver and reduces production of HDL-cholesterol. These adverse changes are associated with hardening and furring-up of the arteries and increased risk of coronary heart disease and stroke.

A pivotal study published in the *American Journal of Clinical Nutrition* in 2000, for example, looked at dietary glycaemic load, carbohydrate intake and risk of coronary heart disease in 75,521 women aged 38 to 63 years who were followed for ten years. The glycaemic load of each person's diet was directly associated with their risk of having a heart attack, after adjusting for age, smoking status, total energy intake and other coronary heart-disease risk factors. Those with the highest glycaemic diet were twice as likely to have a heart attack over the ten-year follow-up period than those following a low glycaemic diet. The link between carbohydrate intake and heart disease risk was most marked in women who were overweight. This study suggests that a high glycaemic load from simple carbohydrates is an independent risk factor for coronary heart disease.

These results have consistently been verified in later meta-analyses and systematic reviews and, while some only showed an association between dietary carbohydrates and heart disease in women, recent Dutch and Finnish studies have shown that a higher total carbohydrate intake, glycaemic index and glycaemic load is associated with a higher risk of heart disease in men compared with lower intakes.

Wholegrains and cognitive function

Brain cells can only use glucose as fuel, not fatty acids. By promoting stable blood glucose levels, wholegrains promote optimum brain function, memory recall and concentration. A cereal breakfast is especially helpful for fuelling the brain as it boosts glucose levels at a crucial time of the day, after the long overnight fast. There appears to be a complex link between what you eat for breakfast and your biorhythms – carbohydrates only have a beneficial, alerting effect on mood if eaten in the morning on waking, and not when you eat them later in the day.

Studies show that schoolchildren who eat a wholegrain cereal breakfast perform better than those who don't, with greater creativity, increased word power and an improved ability to solve problems and learn new information as well as more physical endurance.

Children's exam results can also depend on whether or not they eat breakfast on the day of the test. Among one group of ten-year-olds, those who ate a cereal breakfast made fewer mistakes and worked more quickly in maths tests requiring concentration than those not eating an adequate breakfast. They also showed significant improvements in creativity.

Researchers have also found that adults who regularly eat a cereal breakfast are less depressed, less emotionally distressed and have lower stress levels than those not eating a cereal breakfast. They also have improved memory power, can recall new information more rapidly and have improved concentration and general mental performance. Of course, it's possible that stressed people in stressful jobs are more likely to skip breakfast, but other research supports the fact that you need to eat after your overnight fast to lower secretion of stress hormones and to provide fuel for your brain.

Eating wholegrain cereals for breakfast can also greatly improve performance and endurance for athletes. This is particularly important for prolonged exercise activities such as long-distance running, cycling, triathlon and some team sports.

LESS WELL-KNOWN WHOLEGRAIN FOODS

Hemp pasta is made from flour and oil derived from hemp seed, which is related to sunflower seeds. Hemp seed has similar protein content to soybeans, and hemp-seed oil is a rich source of omega-3 oils and vitamin E.

Red rice (from Camargue or Bhutan) has a distinctive, nutty flavour and a satisfying, chewy texture due to the thin red bran that remains after light milling. It has the same nutritional value as brown rice but cooks twice as quickly.

Wild rice is the seed of a water grass. It is fermented for up to two weeks to make it easier to hull and to improve its nutty flavour. It is often mixed in with brown or red rice for added texture and visual interest.

Quinoa is the seed of a plant related to spinach. It has a slightly smoky flavour and is an excellent source of protein (50 per cent higher than most grains), vitamin E and B-group vitamins plus minerals such as potassium, magnesium, zinc, copper, manganese and folate.

Teff is one of the most ancient grains in the world, and also one of the smallest. Its name even comes from an old word 'teffa' meaning 'lost' because if you drop it on the ground you won't find it again. Teff originated in Ethiopia as a foraged wild grass and was eventually cultivated by the highland Ethiopians. Teff is available in brown and white versions, but both are wholegrain as the kernel is too small to mill easily. Teff supplies more fibre-rich bran and nutritious germ than any other grain, and has a high mineral content including seventeen times more calcium than is found in wholewheat or barley.

Fruit and vegetables: why five a day?

Just about everyone is aware of the recommendations to eat at least five servings of fruit and vegetables per day, but where does this number come from? Why five a day rather than three, four, eight, or even more?

Plant foods are important dietary sources of fibre, phytosterols, isoflavones, carotenoids such as lutein and lycopene, minerals such as selenium and vitamins such as C and E. Most have a low glycaemic index and have beneficial effects on glucose control and insulin sensitivity. This is partly because the soluble fibre they contain helps to slow the absorption of dietary carbohydrates, and partly because their sugars include a blend of glucose and other fruit sugars, such as fructose, that have a lower glycaemic index. Whereas glucose has a GI value of 100, fructose has a GI of just 23.

Researchers have found that people who eat the most fruit and vegetables have a lower risk of developing a number of chronic diseases than those who eat the least. They help to protect against cancer, coronary heart disease, stroke and possibly diabetes. They may also reduce the risk of cataracts, diverticular disease, osteoporosis and obesity.

It is estimated that up to 70 per cent of all cancers are linked to poor diet. A review of over 200 clinical studies found a consistent protective effect of fruit and vegetables against cancers of the stomach, oesophagus, lung, mouth and throat, uterus, pancreas and colon, so the more servings eaten the better. The greatest protection came from eating raw vegetables, onions, garlic, carrots, green vegetables, members of the cabbage family and tomatoes.

People with a high intake of fruit and vegetables have a blood pressure that is around 5 mmHg lower than that of people with the least intakes. In this case, apples, oranges, prunes, grapes, carrots, alfalfa, mushrooms, raw spinach, tofu and celery were the most effective at lowering blood pressure. As a result, they help to protect against stroke. An analysis of eight studies involving over 257,000 people found that eating three to five servings of fruit and vegetables per day reduced the risk of stroke by 11 per cent, compared with those eating fewer than three a day. However, those eating more than five a day had a 26 per cent lower risk. Overall, it seems that each additional portion of fruit you eat per day reduces your risk of stroke by 11 per cent, while each additional portion of vegetables reduces your risk by 3 per cent.

As previously discussed, studies involving over 278,000 people have shown that eating three to five servings of fruit and vegetables per day reduces the risk of coronary heart disease by 7 per cent compared to eating fewer than three servings a day, and that those who eat more than five servings per day enjoy a 17 per cent lower risk.

When researchers in the US looked at the fruit and vegetable consumption of 9,665 adults aged 25 to 75 over 20 years, they found that eating at least five servings of fruit and vegetables per day reduced the risk of women developing Type 2 diabetes by almost 30 per cent – even after taking into account other risk factors such as age, weight, cigarette smoking, blood pressure, cholesterol levels, physical inactivity and alcohol consumption. Vegetables that were the most beneficial for blood glucose control were green leafy vegetables (such as cabbage), beans and some tubers such as Jerusalem artichoke. However, a meta-analysis of data from five large studies involving over 167,000 people found that eating five or more servings of fruit and vegetables per day only reduced the risk of developing Type 2 diabetes by around 4 per cent. This was considerably lower than expected. When the same authors looked at nine studies assessing the antioxidant intake of almost 140,000 people, they found that antioxidant intake, rather than fruit and vegetables, reduced the risk of Type 2 diabetes by 13 per cent, and this was mainly attributed to vitamin E. Reasons for these discrepancies are unclear, and more research is needed.

Overall, however, the evidence suggests that eating five servings of fruit and vegetables per day is good, but that eating *more* than five is considerably better, and that nine to ten servings appears to be the ideal. Potatoes are not classed as a vegetable, but are included in the starchy class of foods.

Each of the following amounts is equivalent to one serving:

- one whole apple, orange, pear, peach, nectarine, kiwi, banana, pomegranate or similar-sized fruit
- two satsumas, plums, apricots, figs, tomatoes or similar-sized fruit
- half a grapefruit, guava, mango, Gaia melon, avocado
- a handful of grapes, cherries, blueberries, strawberries, dates
- a handful of chopped vegetables such as carrots, cabbage, sweetcorn, broccoli florets (and protein-rich pulses such as beans, peas, lentils, chickpeas)
- a small bowl of loosely packed, mixed salad stuff
- a small bowl of vegetable soup
- a wineglassful (100 ml) of fruit or vegetable juice (these only count towards a maximum of one serving per day, as they contain little fibre).

Juice your own

Fruit juices can only count as one serving per day, however much you drink, but although you remove much of the insoluble fibre from fruit or vegetables when juicing, you obtain considerably

more micronutrients than when eating all your fruit and vegetables in their natural raw state. The secret is in their concentration. One hundred millmetres of carrot juice can give you as
much betacarotene as one pound of raw carrots.

Smoothies can count as two servings if they contain at least
two full servings of whole fruit rather than just the juice.

It is worth investing in a juicer to prepare your own delicious
juices. Freshly prepared juice has a creamy texture, a milky hue
and is richer in vitamins and antioxidants than those that have sat
on a shelf or in a fridge for several days. Once you've tasted the
home-made version, you'll never be fully satisfied with those
sold in bottles, cartons or cans again.

Juices can be used to make tasty soups, sauces, drinks or cock-
tails. Lemonade made by mixing a juiced lemon (plus peel) with
sparkling mineral water and a touch of honey is particularly
refreshing.

When buying fruit and vegetables to juice, make sure they're
garden-fresh – as soon as they're harvested, fruit and vegetables start
to deteriorate and their vitamin content drops. If possible, go for
organic ingredients that have not come into contact with artificial
fertilizers or pesticides. Choose firm, plump produce with a good
colour, not mouldy or squidgy ones or those starting to dry out.

Citrus fruit with tough skins need to be peeled before
juicing – but you can process young, unwaxed lemons and limes
intact for extra flavour. Choose seedless grapes and remove the
stalks to avoid bitter flavours. Some fruits, such as bananas and avocados, are difficult for juicers to cope with – they are best mashed
or blended and then stirred into other fruit-juice bases instead.

Virtually any blend of fruit, vegetable or herb is possible –
experiment, and vary the quantities to suit your taste. Try diluting
juices with mineral water for a thirst-quenching drink. Milk and
probiotic yogurt can also be added to smoothies.

Experiment with unusual mixes such as orange and straw-
berry; apple and fig; blueberry and pomegranate; grape and
mango; carrot and watercress; beetroot and tomato; avocado,

carrot and orange; spinach, tomato and celery; tomato, basil and garlic. This variety will provide a wide range of nutrients and broaden your taste buds' experience.

DRIED FRUITS

Although fresh fruit has a low glycaemic load, dried fruits have a concentrated sugar content that gives them a high GL value – in fact, dried figs and dates contain more than 50 per cent sugar. Two or three dried figs or dates therefore make an excellent energy-rich snack, but don't overindulge.

Green leafy vegetables are good sources of vitamin C, carotenoids, folate, fibre, calcium, magnesium, potassium, iron, manganese and selenium (if grown in selenium-rich soils). The iron present in spinach, curly kale and other vegetables is in the non-haem form, which is not so well absorbed as the haem-form iron found in meat. However, the vitamin C present in these green leafy vegetables helps to keep the inorganic form of iron in the ferrous state which, as we have seen, allows for maximum absorption.

Broccoli is one of the most beneficial green vegetables, as it contains a number of protective phytochemicals such as sulphoraphane and the phytoestrogen genistein. Green leafy vegetables and broccoli should be steamed or briefly boiled or stir-fried to help preserve their beneficial nutrients. They can also be eaten raw in salads for optimum nutritional value. Broccoli sprouts are an exceptionally rich source of these phytochemicals and are delicious eaten raw.

Root vegetables

Many people eat just a few types of root vegetable – potatoes, carrots and parsnips, for example. Try to broaden your range, as many less commonly eaten tubers contain a granular form of starch that is more resistant to intestinal enzymes, and therefore has less impact on your blood glucose levels. This 'resistant' starch delivers similar benefits to soluble and insoluble fibre. Jerusalem artichokes, for example, contain an indigestible complex sugar called inulin, which is made up of units of the sugar fructose. This inulin content helps to stabilize glucose levels and is particularly beneficial when combined with foods providing a high glycaemic load. Inulin is also broken down to form fructo-oligo-saccharides, which have a prebiotic effect in the large bowel (see Chapter 6). Similarly, sweet potatoes are orange-fleshed tubers that have a medium glycaemic load rather than the high GL of normal, starchy white potatoes. Sweet potatoes are also a rich source of carotenoids and phytoestrogens.

ORAC scores

Many researchers now believe that coronary heart disease is not so much linked to a high saturated-fat intake but to a lack of dietary antioxidants, which protect circulating fats from oxidation. It is only oxidized LDL-cholesterol that is attacked by circulating scavenger cells and taken into artery walls, where they contribute to the hardening and furring-up process known as atherosclerosis.

Fruit and vegetables are the main dietary source of antioxidants, which include many phytochemicals plus vitamins C and E. Their antioxidant potential can be assessed by measuring their ORAC (Oxygen Radical Absorbance Capacity) score.

HOW THE ORAC TEST WORKS

The ORAC test measures how well the antioxidants in a food prevent the breakdown of a chemical (fluorescein) after it is mixed with a strongly oxidant substance (peroxyl radical). Fluorescein is used because it is luminescent, and the intensity of light it emits decreases as it breaks down. This provides an easy measure of how much fluorescein remains intact at set intervals after mixing the fruit or vegetable extract with the oxidant. A food with a low ORAC value provides little protection and the mixture's luminosity rapidly decreases. A food with a high ORAC value protects the fluorescein from degradation and the sample remains luminescent for longer. By measuring the intensity of fluorescence in the mixture every 35 minutes after adding the oxidant, scientists develop graphs that are compared with the results from different concentrations of a standard antioxidant related to vitamin E (trolox). The final results are given as 'trolox equivalents' or TE. For example, pecan nuts have a high total antioxidant capacity of 179.4 micromol of TE per gram, or 17,940 per 100 g.

Based on surveys of food intake in the US, scientists estimate that the average person obtains around 5,700 ORAC units per day. The optimum ORAC intake is unknown, but it is generally agreed that you need at least 7,000 ORAC units for health, and that intakes of 20,000 ORAC units per day or more are likely to offer greater long-term health benefits. Table 13 shows the ORAC score of selected fruit and vegetables.

The fruit and vegetables you select therefore have a major impact on your antioxidant intake. If you select five servings made up of blueberries, black plums, pomegranate, blackberries and a red apple, you can obtain over 40,000 ORAC units in a single day. But if your five servings comprise a banana, slice of watermelon, lettuce, cauliflower plus a tomato and cucumber salad, you would obtain little more than 2,000 ORAC units – even though you met the recommended five-a-day requirement.

Balancing your intake of foods with high, medium and low ORAC scores can optimize the antioxidant potential of your diet. The higher a fruit or vegetable's ORAC score, the higher its ability to neutralize free radicals (the molecular

Table 13 ORAC score per serving of selected fruit
and vegetables

Fruit/vegetable	ORAC score* per average serving
Dark chocolate cocoa solids	41,588
Low-bush blueberries	13,427
Pomegranate	10,500
Cranberries	8,983
Blackberries	7,701
Prunes	7,291
Raspberries	6,058
Red Delicious apple	5,900
Golden Delicious apple	3,685
Lemons/limes	3,378
Oranges (navel)	2,540
Red grapes	2,016
Green grapes	1,789
Banana	1,037
Tomatoes	415
Cauliflower	324
Iceberg lettuce	144
Cucumber	60

* ORAC score = micromol of TE.

fragments that damage cells through a chemical process known as oxidation).

As well as supplying antioxidants, fruit and vegetables provide other important phytochemicals and nutrients including vitamins, minerals, trace elements and fibre. Ideally, the majority of the five to ten servings of fruit and vegetables you eat per day (e.g. three out of five, or seven out of ten) should be in the form of vegetables rather than fruit, even though vegetables tend to have a lower ORAC score. This is because vegetables tend to contain less water, so are a more concentrated source of nutrients, and less sugar as well as more fibre.

A number of herbs and spices have a surprisingly high ORAC score, too, even though you only eat them in small amounts. The following table gives their ORAC values per gram – not per 100 g as in the table above. Adding just one gram of black pepper to a meal gives you an additional 301 ORAC units, while a gram of cinnamon supplies 2,675 ORAC units.

Use the antioxidant-rich herbs and spices shown in Table 14 to replace salt for added flavour and nutritional value.

Table 14 ORAC score per gram of selected culinary herbs and spices

Spice/herb	ORAC score* per gram
Cloves	3,144
Cinnamon	2,675
Oregano	2,001
Turmeric	1,592
Nutmeg	1,572
Parsley	743
Saffron	530
Curry powder	485
Black peppercorns	301
Ginger powder	288

(*Continued*)

Table 14 Cont'd

Spice/herb	ORAC score* per gram
Thyme	274
Chilli powder	236
Mint	139
Garlic	54

*ORAC score = micromol of TE.

Pulses

Pulses, also known as beans or legumes, are plant seeds of varying size, shape and colour that are harvested within a pod. They may be eaten fresh, or dried and reconstituted by soaking in water before cooking and eating. In agricultural terms, though, the word 'pulse' tends to be reserved for crops harvested for use as a dry seed. This excludes green beans and green peas, which are considered vegetable crops. Some classifications also exclude crops grown for oil extraction such as soybeans and peanuts – even though both are seeds extracted from a pod and therefore would normally be classified as a legume (in which seeds form in a pod, for example peas, beans). In practical terms, peanuts eaten as a snack food, rather than used to extract groundnut oil, are usually considered along with nuts, as in the section below.

Pulses are a good source of vitamins and minerals (especially potassium, calcium, magnesium, iron and zinc) as well as trace elements. Although almost a fifth of their energy content is in the form of carbohydrate, it is in a complex, slowly digested form, and so they have a low glycaemic load.

Within the food pyramid, pulses can be counted as part of the vegetables group and consumed frequently – several portions per week as a vegetable selection. They can also be counted as a protein source as part of the meat, poultry, fish, dry beans, eggs and nuts group. This is because pulses are a good source of protein of comparable nutritional value to fish, poultry and meat. Most pulses except soy, however, lack some essential amino acids. Chickpeas and other pulses are therefore best combined with other plant foods and wholegrains such as brown rice and wholemeal bread to provide a balanced amino acid intake. As a general rule, vegetarians can obtain a balanced protein intake by eating a combination of five parts rice to one part beans. Pulses are also a rich source of phytochemicals, especially isoflavones and other antioxidants that give them a high ORAC score, as shown in Table 15.

Soybeans are an excellent source of protein, which is comparable in its amino acid content to meat. They are also a good source of calcium, potassium, magnesium, iron, zinc, manganese, B-group vitamins, folate and selenium. Soy and soy products such as tofu, miso and soy milk also provide additional health

Table 15 ORAC score per serving of selected pulses

Pulses	*ORAC score* per average serving*
Red kidney beans	13,259
Pinto beans	11,864
Red lentils	7,325
Soybeans	5,764
Black beans	4,181
Chickpeas (garbanzo)	3,022
Navy beans	2,573
Black-eyed peas	2,258

*ORAC score = micromol of TE.

benefits in the form of isoflavone phytoestrogens (genistein, daidzein and glycitein). A diet that is low in saturated fat and cholesterol, and which includes 25 g soy protein per day, can significantly reduce the risk of coronary heart disease. As a guide, 60 g of soy protein provides 45 mg isoflavones, which is one of the reasons why populations with high intakes, such as Japan, have an unusually low risk of heart attack.

Lentils are a good source of phytoestrogen lignans, and contain useful amounts of isoflavones. They also contain beneficial amounts of potassium, magnesium, iron, copper, zinc, selenium and B-group vitamins.

Red kidney beans have an exceptionally high ORAC score due largely to their antioxidant pigments. However, they must be boiled rapidly for at least 15 minutes, then simmered until thoroughly cooked. This denatures substances (lectins) which can otherwise lead to indigestion and symptoms similar to food poisoning. Soaking beans overnight reduces cooking times, and also helps to deactivate the indigestible sugars that are fermented by bacteria to produce intestinal wind. Kidney beans provide twice as much fibre as green beans. They are also a good source of potassium and contain useful amounts of folate, calcium, magnesium, iron, zinc and selenium.

Nuts and seeds

Nuts are the edible kernels of hard-shelled seeds. These, and edible plant seeds with softer shells, supply a concentrated source of energy which is mostly supplied in the form of fat and protein and means that they have a low glycaemic index. They are also a good source of fibre, typically providing around 6 g fibre per 100 g.

The types of fats found in nuts are nutritionally valuable oils containing a high percentage of beneficial monounsaturated and polyunsaturated essential fatty acids. For example, macadamia-nut oil is 81 per cent monounsaturated, hemp-seed oil is 80 per cent polyunsaturated and sesame-seed oil is 39 per cent mono-unsaturated and 45 per cent polyunsaturated.

Oil from flaxseed (also known as linseed) is an unusually rich source of the omega-3 essential fatty acid alpha-linolenic acid (ALA). It also contains the omega-6 essential fatty acid linoleic acid, so its ratio of beneficial, anti-inflammatory omega-3s com-pared to the pro-inflammatory omega-6s is around 3:1. In con-trast, oil from the seeds of the non-drug strain of cannabis, known as the hemp plant, has an omega-3/omega-6 ratio of 1:3 – the opposite to that found in flaxseed oil, which might be expected to promote inflammation in the body. However, a considerable amount of omega-6 is in the form of gamma-linolenic acid (GLA) – the one omega-6 that actually has an anti-inflammatory action. Other nuts and seeds contain a variable blend of omega-6s and omega-3s.

Nuts are also a rich source of vitamins, minerals, trace ele-ments and antioxidant phytochemicals that give them a high ORAC score (see Table 16).

Almonds contain vitamin E and flavanol antioxidants, which prevent oxidation of LDL-cholesterol so that it is more readily carried back to the liver for processing. This means that eating a handful of almonds per day (about 23 kernels) can lower 'bad' LDL-cholesterol by 5 per cent and increase 'good' HDL-cholesterol by 6 per cent. And in practical terms, researchers estimate that eating a handful of almonds per day can improve your cholesterol balance enough to reduce your risk of a heart attack or stroke by around 20 per cent.

Brazil nuts are the richest dietary source of selenium, which plays an important immune role and provides antioxidant protec-tion against cancer. Research involving over 1,110 Finnish males also suggests that selenium helps to protect against stroke. Those with the lowest selenium levels were almost four times more

Table 16 ORAC score of selected nuts

Nut	ORAC score* per 30 g serving
Pecans	5,095
Walnuts	3,846
Hazelnuts	2,739
Pistachios	2,267
Almonds	1,265
Peanuts	899
Cashews	567
Macadamias	481
Brazil nuts	403
Pine kernels	204

*ORAC score = micromol of TE.

likely to experience a stroke than those with the highest levels. Whether or not it also protects against coronary heart disease remains uncertain, although it is possible that selenium may reduce the risk of non-fatal heart attack.

Macadamia nuts and *hazelnuts* are among the richest dietary sources of monounsaturated fats. As well as lowering 'bad' LDL-cholesterol levels, monounsaturated fat has an anti-inflammatory action and a beneficial effect on immunity.

Peanuts are a source of the antioxidant phytochemical resveratrol – also found in red wine – which is believed to protect against atherosclerosis and coronary heart disease. Unfortunately, peanuts are often eaten roasted or salted, which detracts from their nutritional value – eat them fresh and unsalted for maximum health benefits.

Walnuts are a good source of omega-3 essential oils that have a beneficial effect on cholesterol balance as well as reducing inflammation. They are also a good source of antioxidants such as vitamin E and selenium. Research suggests that regular consumption of walnuts can lower 'bad' LDL-cholesterol enough to reduce the risk of coronary heart disease by 30 to 50 per cent and increase lifespan by an estimated five to ten years.

Aim to eat around 30 g of nuts or seeds daily either as a healthy snack, or added to muesli or bread and sprinkled onto salads and other meals. Buy them fresh, little and often, for maximum freshness, from a shop with a rapid turnover.

Milk and dairy products

Milk is an important source of calcium for healthy bones and teeth. Dairy products that retain their calcium content are included in this group, but those that consist mostly of milk fats (cream and butter) are not, as these provide energy in the form of fat with little additional nutritional value. The nutrient content of important members of this group is shown in Table 17.

Most people would benefit from obtaining three servings of these products per day, which should ideally be low-fat or fat-free such as skimmed or semi-skimmed milk, low-fat natural fromage frais or yogurt, cottage cheese and just small amounts of fat-dense hard cheese (40 g or 1½ oz).

Lactose intolerance

A surprising number of people are intolerant of the milk sugar, lactose, which is naturally present in sheep, cows' and goats' milk in similar quantities (around 10 g per glass). Worldwide, lactose intolerance affects 95 per cent of people of Asian origin, over

Table 17 Nutrient content of selected dairy products per 100 g

Food	Carbohydrate (as sugars)	Protein	Fat	Energy	Calcium
Skimmed milk	4 g	3 g	0.2 g	32 kcal	122 mg
Semi-skimmed milk	5 g	3 g	1.7 g	46 kcal	120 mg
Whole milk	4.5 g	3 g	4 g	66 kcal	118 mg
Cheddar cheese	0	25 g	35 g	416 kcal	739 mg
Brie soft cheese	0	20 g	29 g	343 kcal	256 mg
Cottage cheese (low-fat)	3 g	13 g	1.5 g	79 kcal	485 mg

75 per cent of Afro-Caribbean people and 50 per cent of those from South America. North-Western Europeans and those with European ancestry such as white North Americans, however, are less likely to be affected. Normally, all mammals produce the lactase enzyme needed to break down milk sugar (lactose) whilst being breastfed. After weaning, lactase enzyme secretion reduces then stops in preparation for following an adult diet that, traditionally, has consisted of meat, grains, vegetables and fruit but no dairy products. A few thousand years ago, however, a genetic mutation occurred in the lactase gene so that lactose production persisted. This is thought to have arisen in Europe within a population of dairy farmers. Retaining lactase activity provided a survival advantage as it allowed the continued consumption of nutritionally rich cows' milk – especially when other foods were scarce. It was passed on as a dominant genetic trait (i.e. only one copy of the gene that allows lactase persistence is needed for someone to continue tolerating milk into adulthood). This mutation – and similar ones arising spontaneously elsewhere – quickly spread among populations in Northern Europe and Scandinavia,

and also included some nomadic peoples travelling to the Middle East and Africa.

Lactose is a disaccharide made up of two sugars, galactose and glucose, joined together. Lactose is digested by an enzyme, lactase, secreted by cells within the lining of the small intestines. This separates the galactose and glucose, which are then absorbed. When insufficient amounts of lactase are produced, however, lactose stays within the gut to reach the large intestines, where it is fermented by bowel bacteria. This can produce symptoms of nausea, bloating, audible bowel sounds (borborygmi), wind, cramping abdominal pains and diarrhoea.

People who suspect they are lactose intolerant may find that cutting lactose from their diet and using milk alternatives can alleviate the symptoms. Low-lactose cows' milk is available, containing less than 1 g lactose per glass, while milks made from soy, rice and nuts are lactose-free. Yogurt made from cows' milk also has a low lactose content, as bacterial fermentation breaks the lactose down. Alternatively, lactase drops can be added to any drink to replenish the missing enzyme.

If you are avoiding milk products because of lactose intolerance, you will need to ensure an adequate intake of calcium from alternative sources such as calcium-enriched soy milk, eggs, green leafy vegetables, whitebait, tinned salmon and sardines (which include soft bones), pulses, nuts and seeds.

Fish

As shown in Table 18, fish are an excellent source of protein. Oily fish such as herring, salmon, mackerel and pilchards are also a rich source of long-chain, omega-3 polyunsaturated fatty acids and vitamin D. The flesh of white fish, such as cod and tinned tuna (which has been processed) contain very little omega-3 oil, however.

Table 18 Nutrient content of selected fish

Food	Protein per 100 g	Fat per 100 g	Total long-chain omega-3 per 100 g	Vitamin D per 100 g	Energy per 100 g
Herring	18 g	13 g	1.3 g	19 mcg	190 kcal
Salmon, fresh	18 g	12 g	2.2 g	16 mcg	182 kcal
Salmon, canned in brine (drained)	24 g	7 g	1.6 g	9 mcg	153 kcal
Mackerel	19 g	16 g	1.9 g	8 mcg	220 kcal
Kippers	18 g	18 g	2.6 g	8 mcg	229 kcal
Pilchards (canned in tomato sauce)	17 g	8 g	2.6 g	14 mcg	144 kcal
Tuna, fresh	23 g	5 g	1.3 g	1 mcg	144 kcal
Tuna (canned in oil, drained)	27 g	9 g	0.4 g	3 mcg	189 kcal
Cod	18 g	<1 g	0.3 g	trace	80 kcal
Haddock	19 g	<1 g	0.2 g	trace	81 kcal
Plaice	17 g	<1 g	0.3 g	trace	79 kcal

The omega-3 fatty acids found in fish oils are the long-chain docosahexaenoic acid (DHA) and eicosapentaenoic acid (EPA), which are derived from the microalgae on which the fish feed. These omega-3 fatty acids are used in the body to make substances (series 3 prostaglandins and series 5 leukotrienes) that have an anti-inflammatory action, and help to protect against inflammatory conditions such as arthritis, asthma, eczema and coronary heart disease which is linked with low-grade inflammation in the artery walls.

Fish oils and heart disease

Research has shown that omega-3 fish oils help to reduce blood pressure, to lower raised circulating triglyceride levels, to prevent abnormal blood clotting and protect against abnormal heart rhythms (especially in heart muscle receiving a poor blood supply). As a result, even modest increases in dietary intakes of oily fish can help to prevent a fatal heart attack. In those who have already had a heart attack, increasing consumption of fish significantly reduces the chance of a second heart attack and, if one does occur, the chances of dying from this second heart attack. An intake of at least 1 g omega-3 fish oils per day from eating oily fish twice a week or from pharmaceutical-grade supplements has consistently been shown to reduce the risk of sudden cardiac death by 40 to 45 per cent. As a result, both the American Heart Association and the European Society of Cardiology recommend a daily intake of 1 g long-chain, omega-3 fish oils as a preventive measure in those at risk of coronary heart disease. In fact, eating oily fish at least twice a week can lower your risk of a fatal heart attack more than following a low-fat, high-fibre diet. Although it is worth noting that the protective effects of oily fish are seen after only six months. After two years, those on a high fish diet are almost a third less likely to die from coronary heart disease than those eating the least amount of fish.

Fish oils and stroke

People who regularly eat oily fish are less likely to die from stroke than those who do not. A meta-analysis of data from six studies suggests that eating any fish on a weekly basis reduces the risk of stroke by 12 per cent, with each additional portion reducing the risk by another 2 per cent per serving per week.

Fish oils and arthritis

For those with arthritic joint pains, omega-3 fish oils lower the level of inflammatory chemicals and thus reduce pain in a similar way to that of non-steroidal anti-inflammatory drugs, as they inhibit inflammatory enzymes (COX-1 and COX-2) to reduce joint pain and swelling. Consequently, a number of studies show that taking fish-oil supplements can reduce the need for taking non-steroidal anti-inflammatory drug (NSAID) painkillers. High intakes of 3 g to 6 g EPA and DHA are needed per day, however, for a good anti-inflammatory effect in joints.

To obtain this level of intake from eating fish alone is an unrealistic target. The average adult following a Western-style diet only eats one-third of a portion of oily fish per week, and two out of three adults eat no oily fish at all. Average intakes of the long-chain omega-3s EPA and DHA therefore average just 1 g per week. In addition, some government agencies suggest limiting intakes of deep-sea fish to reduce exposure to marine pollutants such as mercury (linked to impaired neurological development), dioxins and PCBs, both of which are linked to reduced immunity, reduced fertility and some cancers.

LIMITING INTAKES

In the UK, there are now limits on the maximum recommended intake of oily fish, and some white fish and crabmeat.

Oily fish Although you should eat at least one portion (140 g) of oily fish a week, boys, men and women past reproductive age should eat no more than four portions of oily fish per week to reduce exposure to marine pollutants such as mercury, dioxins and PCBs (polychlorinated biphenyls) that can build up in the body. Girls and women of childbearing age should eat no more than two portions of oily fish a week as these marine pollutants may affect the development of a baby in the future.

Canned tuna If you are trying for a baby, or are pregnant, do not have more than four cans of tuna (140 g drained weight each) a week because of its mercury content. There is no limit for breast-feeding. Canned tuna is not classed as an oily fish, so you can eat this in addition to your maximum two portions of oily fish per week (as long as you don't have fresh tuna).

White fish Children, pregnant women and women who are trying to become pregnant should also avoid shark, swordfish and marlin. Other adults should have no more than one portion of shark, swordfish or marlin per week. This is because they can contain more mercury than other fish.

Other white fish that may contain similar levels of certain pollutants as oily fish are sea bream; sea bass; turbot; halibut; rock salmon (also known as dogfish, flake, huss, rigg or rock eel).

Anyone who regularly eats a lot of fish should avoid eating these five fish but may otherwise safely eat as many portions of white fish per week as they like, and ideally should aim for at least two.

Crab Avoid eating the brown meat from crabs too often. There is no need to limit the amount of white crabmeat that you eat.

Omega-3 fish-oil supplements are an effective way to increase your intakes of EPA and DHA as they are screened to ensure low levels of pollutants. If you eat no oily fish, six high-strength capsules per day are needed to provide 3 g omega-3s, the ideal amount for a noticeable anti-inflammatory effect in those with painful, osteoarthritic joints. If you eat two portions of an oily fish such as salmon per week, however, you would only need four high-strength capsules per day to obtain the same level of intake. If you do not have painful joints, but wish to obtain the cardioprotective effects of fish oils, then a 1 g high–strength capsule per day is sufficient.

FISH-OIL SUPPLEMENTS

Standard fish-oil capsules typically provide 180 mg EPA and 120 mg DHA per 1 g capsule (a ratio of 3:2).

High-strength oils contain around 310 mg EPA and 210 mg DHA.

Cod liver oil naturally contains 170 mg total EPA plus DHA per 1 g capsule.

Select a pharmaceutical-grade fish-oil supplement to ensure they are free from marine pollutants. Those offered in the triglyceride (TG) form are most easily absorbed and used in the body.

If choosing to take cod liver oil, those described as high- or extra-high strength provide the highest amount of omega-3 fatty acids. If taking a multivitamin as well, check that the total amounts of vitamin A and D do not exceed recommended doses – vitamin A is best limited to less than 1,500 mcg per day; vitamin D's upper safe level is 25 mcg daily.

NB Women who are pregnant should avoid cod liver oil supplements (due to their high vitamin A content) and select DHA-rich oils especially designed for pregnancy.

Fish oils and depression

DHA plays an important structural role within brain–cell membranes, improving their fluidity so that messages are passed on more rapidly from one cell to another. EPA is involved in cell signalling and also improves communication between brain cells. Studies suggest that populations who eat fish infrequently have higher levels of depression compared with those who eat fish regularly, and adding fish oils (2 g per day) to the usual drug treatment for depression has been shown to improve symptoms within two weeks, compared with placebo.

A recent meta-analysis of 15 randomized placebo-controlled trials involving 916 people, published in the *Journal of Clinical Psychiatry*, found that EPA-rich fish-oil supplements were effective against primary depression.

There is some evidence that fish oils may help to improve painful periods, dyslexia and protect against age-related macular degeneration. In children with attention-deficit hyperactivity disorders, fish oils may help to improve cognitive scores and general behaviour, although this is controversial.

FORTIFIED OMEGA-3S

Healthy staple foods such as margarines, bread and even milk are often fortified with omega-3 oils to help boost intakes in those who do not eat much fish. However, few of these are fortified with the long-chain omega-3s (EPA and DHA). Many of these products contain only tiny amounts of added omega-3s, usually of the short-chain variety (ALA) derived from vegetable oils. Less than 5 per cent of these are converted on to EPA in the body, and less than 0.5 per cent are transformed into DHA.

Fish oils and diabetes

In the early days of fish-oil research, it was suggested that they may increase blood sugar levels in people with Type 2 diabetes. However, several large-scale analyses have now concluded that taking a fish-oil supplement has no real effect on glucose control in this group. On the contrary, studies now show that omega-3 fish oils can boost glucose tolerance as well as improving other heart-disease risk factors associated with diabetes. In fact, some studies suggest that increased dietary intake of omega-3 fish oils with reduced intake of saturated fat may lower the risk of someone with impaired glucose tolerance progressing to Type 2 diabetes. If you have diabetes, and choose to take any food supplements, including fish oils, always monitor your glucose levels closely.

In summary

Most people would benefit from increasing their intake of long-chain omega-3s and cutting back on their intake of omega-6s to obtain a better balance of polyunsaturated fats.

Aim to eat more omega-3 rich oily fish (two to four portions per week) such as mackerel, herring, salmon, trout, sardines, pilchards, fresh tuna (not tinned), wild game meat (such as venison and buffalo), grass-fed beef and omega-3 enriched eggs. At the same time, cut out excess omega-6s by consuming less omega-6 vegetable oils (safflower oil, grapeseed oil, sunflower oil, corn oil, cottonseed oil or soybean oil) and replace with healthier oils such as rapeseed, olive, walnut or macadamia oils. Other omega-6 rich foods to avoid (or at least consume only in moderation) are margarines based on omega-6 oils such as sunflower or safflower oil, convenience foods, fast foods and manufactured goods such as cakes, sweets and pastries.

Meat

Meat is an important source of protein as it supplies all the essential and non-essential amino acids. It is also a good source of iron. As explained in Chapter 2, although meat fat is usually classified as 'bad' saturated fat, it is also an excellent source of healthy monounsaturated fat, which it often supplies more than any other source. Table 19 shows the relative amounts of saturated and monounsaturated fat found in lean, raw cuts of various meats. Meat is also a source of dietary, preformed cholesterol.

Table 19 **Nutrient content of selected meats**

Meat (raw, lean)	Total fat per 100 g	% saturated	% Mono- unsaturated	Omega-3s per 100 g	Cholesterol
Beef	4.3 g	39%	44%	20 mg	58 mg
Pork	4 g	35%	38%	20 mg	63 mg
Lamb	8 g	44%	39%	78 mg	74 mg
Venison	7.1 g	48%	18%	104 mg	80 mg
Rabbit	5.5 g	38%	24%	90 mg	53 mg
Duck	6.5 g	31%	49%	80 mg	110 mg
Chicken white meat	1.1 g	27%	45%	40 mg	70 mg
Chicken dark meat	2.8 g	29%	46%	110 mg	105 mg
Turkey light meat	0.8 g	38%	38%	40 mg	57 mg
Turkey dark meat	2.5 g	32%	40%	90 mg	86 mg

White meats such as chicken and turkey tend to have a lower fat content than red meats, but sizeable amounts of fat (and calories) can be avoided by trimming meats of all visible fat before cooking. As most of the fat in poultry is in the skin, this is also easily removed either before or after cooking.

Meat is also an important source of micronutrients, especially iron, zinc, B vitamins, vitamin D and selenium, as well as supplying useful amounts of magnesium, copper, cobalt, phosphorus and chromium.

There are concerns that cooking meat in a way that crisps it (frying, chargrilling and barbecuing), and consuming processed meats, may increase your exposure to chemicals (N-nitroso-compounds) that are linked with bowel cancer. However, studies are inconclusive and these findings may have more to do with high-fat diets and the cooking methods (overcooking or char-ring meat) rather than the meat itself. Even so, it is generally recommended that you limit your intake of red meat to no more than 500 g cooked red meat per week (equivalent to 70 g, or half a small beefsteak every day). Average intakes in the UK are around 96 g red meat per day for men, and 57 g red meat for women.

For some people, especially men, following these guidelines means cutting back on portion sizes and exchanging meat-based meals with fish, bean-based vegetarian meals and swapping some red meat for white meats such as chicken and turkey.

The Mediterranean diet

Researchers became interested in the Mediterranean diet when it was noted that people living in Greece, Crete and southern Italy had unusually low risks for developing coronary heart disease, cancer and other diet-related illnesses such as Type 2 dia-betes. These populations also had one of the highest adult life expectancies in the world.

When researchers looked at the results of a number of studies investigating high blood pressure, cardiovascular disease, obesity and cancer, they found that individuals who reported eating foods consistent with the Mediterranean diet were between 10 and 20 per cent less likely to die over the course of the studies from any cause, including heart disease and cancer.

The Mediterranean diet combines relatively large amounts of vegetables, fruit, olive oil, fish, garlic, wholegrains, beans, nuts, seeds, bread and potatoes with a relatively low intake of red meat and a moderate consumption of red wine. Overall, it provides a total fat content of 25 to 35 per cent with a low saturated-fat intake of 8 per cent or less of energy intake. Good intakes of omega-3 fatty acids, monounsaturated fats, dietary antioxidants, vitamins, minerals and phytochemicals are also present.

In the Lyon Diet Heart Study, one group of people who had experienced a heart attack were asked to follow a Mediterranean-style diet, while a similar group were asked to follow a 'prudent Western-style diet'. Those following the Mediterranean diet were significantly less likely to have a second heart attack than those following the 'prudent Western diet'. The protective effects were so striking that the study was terminated after 27 months (rather than the planned five years). It was thought unethical not to advise those in the control group also to follow a Mediterranean way of eating which was associated with a 70 per cent reduction in death from any cause.

Researchers have since discovered that following a Mediterranean-style diet influences the activity of genes involved in the production of inflammatory chemicals, the formation of scavenger cells which engulf oxidized LDL-cholesterol (to become trapped in artery walls – see Chapter 2) and abnormal blood clotting. Together, these benefits reduce the development and progression of hardening and furring-up of the arteries (atherosclerosis).

Researchers estimate that following a traditional Mediterranean diet could prevent over 80 per cent of heart attacks, 70 per cent of strokes and reduce the incidence of Type 2 diabetes by 90 per cent – as long as you also take regular exercise and refrain from smoking cigarettes. Some evidence also suggests that following a Mediterranean diet may slow the onset of age-related cognitive decline by promoting healthy arteries and blood flow to the brain.

It is relatively easy to start obtaining the health benefits of the Mediterranean diet. Information is available on the website www.oldwayspt.org.

In the Lyon Diet Heart Study, participants were simply advised to:

- eat more bread, more root vegetables, green vegetables and more fish
- eat less beef, lamb and pork (replace with poultry)
- have no day without fruit
- replace butter and cream with a margarine high in alpha-linoleic acid
- cut back on other types of food including biscuits, cakes, sweets and desserts, which are easily replaced with fruit.

To add to that advice, I would suggest selecting wholegrain bread and wholegrain cereals rather than 'white' versions, using olive oil rather than other cooking/dressing oils and consuming wine in low to moderate amounts (one to two glasses per day for men, and one glass per day for women).

Healthy cooking methods

By cooking your food in the healthiest ways possible, the fat content of your diet can be minimized and the nutrient content optimized. Preferred methods of cooking include:

- steaming
- grilling with only a light brushing of olive oil plus herbs, lemon juices and spices for flavour
- dry baking
- baking *en papillotte* (wrapping in greaseproof paper or silver foil) so that food steams gently in its own parcel
- boiling with only the minimal amount of water and no added salt or bicarbonate of soda

- poaching in home-made vegetable stock (court bouillon)
- dry- (stir-) frying using a light brushing of olive oil
- if roasting meat, placing the meat on a rack within the roasting pan so that all the juices and fats drain away
- when roasting chicken, using a glass funnel roaster onto which you prop the chicken vertically in the oven. All the fats then drain off so you are left with beautifully flavoured, low-fat meat and virtually fat-free skin
- when making gravy, reusing the water your vegetables were cooked in to reclaim lost micronutrients.

Checking labels

When buying pre-packaged products, it's a good idea to get into the habit of checking labels. As well as helping you compare prices and pack weights, these tell you the nutritional value of what you are buying with ingredients listed in descending order of weight. Most labels show the amount of calories, fat, sugar, fibre and sodium or salt in a product, and may display them per 100 g and per serving.

In the UK, manufacturers have adopted front-of-pack food labelling, which focuses on fat, saturates, sugars and salt – the main dietary ingredients that you need to limit to reduce your risk of heart disease. Two main approaches are used – either the traffic-light or the GDA (Guideline Daily Amount) systems.

The traffic light system

This system of labelling shows you at a glance whether a food contains a high (red), medium (amber), or low (green) amount of fat, saturates, sugar or salt. The label tells you how much of these substances is present in a given serving, stated in grams. If that part of the label is red, the amount present is higher than desirable for regular consumption, and best reserved to eat occasionally, in small amounts. If that part of the food label has an amber background, the food is neither high nor low in that substance and is mostly an OK choice – but 'green' is ideal as it suggests the food is low in that substance.

The traffic-light system isn't foolproof, as a food such as fresh salmon, which is high in healthy oils, will have its fat content highlighted on a red background, and yet most of us would benefit from eating more oily fish. In addition, the traffic-light system doesn't show you how much of a substance is present as a percentage of the daily recommended amount.

Guideline Daily Amounts (GDAs)

Guideline Daily Amounts focus on calories, sugar, fat, saturates and salt. These show you at a glance how much of each substance is present in a portion of the food and the percentage of an adult's guideline daily amount it represents (based on a healthy weight, average activity level and no special dietary requirements for females, and assuming a calorie need of 2,000 kcals per day). Of course everyone is different, and men will have different average GDAs to women, but they still give you a good idea of what's in the food you're buying and what you are eating. So if you're trying to cut back on salt or fat, compare labels in similar items and select the product that provides the lowest percentage of your GDA. For more information on how to use GDAs, visit the www.whatsinsideguide.com.

Ideally you want to aim for products that are both low-fat and low-sugar – but be careful, as many low-fat products are actually quite high in sugar content. When checking labels, useful benchmarks are that per 100 g food (or per serving if a serving is less than 100 g):

2 g of sugar or less is **a little** sugar
10 g of sugar or more is **a lot** of sugar.

3 g of total fat or less is **a little** fat
20 g of total fat or more is **a lot** of fat

1 g of saturated fat or less is **a little** saturated fat
5 g of saturated fat or more is **a lot** of saturated fat

0.1 g sodium or less is **a little** sodium
0.5 g sodium or more is **a lot** of sodium

9

Omnivores, piscivores, vegetarians and vegans

Although meat is an important food group, many people choose to avoid it. Most non-meat-eaters are very food-aware and know how to obtain a healthy, balanced diet. As a result, vegetarians tend to enjoy some protection against common Western diseases such as obesity, gallstones, diverticular disease, high blood pressure, diabetes, coronary heart disease and even cancer (especially of the lung and colon). These beneficial effects may partly be due to other healthy lifestyle choices such as the fact that vegetarians are statistically more likely to take regular exercise and less likely to smoke cigarettes or drink excessive amounts of alcohol than meat eaters.

However, a bad vegetarian diet is just as harmful to health as a bad omnivore diet. Some people switch to vegetarianism by simply removing meat (and sometimes dairy products) from their diet without taking steps to substitute other dietary sources of important nutrients. In some cases, vegetarians – especially teenagers and those living alone – have been found to live on a diet of pastries, cakes, quiches, chips, peanuts and crisps while eating hardly any fruit or vegetables at all. Such a regime will quickly increase the risk of future problems such as osteoporosis, anaemia and other dietary deficiency diseases.

Degrees of meat avoidance

Some people prefer not to eat certain meats from certain animals (e.g. veal, pork). This may be due to personal food dislikes, or for religious, cultural or ethical reasons. For example, many Hindus, particularly Brahmins, are vegetarian, but those that do eat meat avoid beef, as the cow is sacred in their religion. Similarly, those who follow the Jewish or Muslim faiths abstain from eating pork. In the West, some people who are not vegetarian prefer to avoid veal and/or cage-reared chickens as they object to the conditions in which these livestock are reared. Their remaining diet includes other meats and fish, and no additional risk of a nutrient deficiency is incurred.

Some people prefer not to eat red meat or poultry, but do eat fish and dairy produce. This is a healthy-eating option and there is little additional risk of nutritional deficiency. This way of eating is sometimes described as fishitarian, pescatarian or piscivorean.

A large number of people choose not to eat meat or fish but do eat milk and eggs. This is described as ovo–lacto vegetarianism. Lacto vegetarianism is similar, except eggs are also excluded. Those following this way of eating need to ensure that they obtain alternative sources of the important micronutrients found in meat and fish, such as iron, zinc and vitamin B12.

Diets that exclude all meat and dairy products derived from animals (which may include honey) is known as veganism. Some vegan diets emphasize eating only organically grown foods, with no chemical additives or salt. Problems arise because vitamin B12 deficiency is almost universal among vegans without regular supplementation. Other nutrients of which intakes are likely to be low when following a vegan diet include iron, calcium and zinc.

Avoiding nutrient deficiencies

Meat is a source of a number of important nutrients including protein, iron and vitamin B12. Vegetarians, and particularly vegans, must therefore obtain these nutrients from other dietary sources.

Protein

It is unlikely that vegetarians will be deficient in protein. Even people who eat meat or fish daily get half their protein from non-meat sources such as cereals (mainly bread and pasta), milk products, fish and eggs. Vegans, however, will need to ensure they consume pulses or grains at each meal.

Vitamin B12

Vitamin B12 is chiefly derived from animal sources, and most vegetarians are aware of the need to watch their intake of this important nutrient. Several sources of vitamin B12 are suitable for vegetarians. Non-meat sources of vitamin B12 include eggs, milk, yogurt and cheese. Vegans should consider supplements derived from vitamin B12-enriched yeasts, preparations made by bacterial fermentation and extracts derived from microalgae.

Iron

Eggs are a good non-meat source of haem iron, but vegetables contain the less absorbable non-haem iron. This is partly compensated for by their higher intake of vitamin C, which increases absorption of non-haem iron by keeping it in the ferrous rather than the ferric form. Some types of plant fibre, especially phytates, decrease the absorption of minerals such as iron, zinc and calcium. Ovo-lacto vegetarians, especially women with heavy periods or who are pregnant, need to ensure they obtain enough iron.

Non-meat sources of iron include brewer's yeast, wheatgerm, wholemeal bread, fortified breakfast cereals, prunes and other dried fruit, green leafy vegetables, parsley, cocoa and curry powder.

Over-boiling vegetables decreases their iron availability by up to 20 per cent. Vitamin C increases the absorption of inorganic iron, while tannin-containing drinks (e.g. tea) decrease it. Coffee can reduce iron absorption by up to 39 per cent if drunk within an hour of eating.

Calcium

Cutting out dairy products can result in a lack of calcium. Some types of fibre (phytates from wheat in unleavened bread – chapattis, for example) bind calcium in the bowel to form an insoluble, non-absorbable salt. In a high-fibre vegetarian diet, which speeds the passage of food through the bowels, the amount of calcium absorbed is also reduced. Vegans, with their traditional preference for wholemeal bread, could try calcium-enriched soy milk and include some white bread in their diet to counter the effects of their exceptionally high-fibre intake. Non-meat sources of calcium include: milk, cheese, yogurt, fromage frais, soy milk, green leafy vegetables, nuts, seeds, pulses, bread made from fortified flour, fortified cereals and eggs.

Vitamin D

Vitamin D is essential for the absorption of calcium from the small intestine but it is not found in many vegetarian foods, and that which is present in plants is in the form of vitamin D2, which is less well absorbed and used in the body than the animal form, vitamin D3. Some vitamin D3 can be synthesized in the body by the action of sunlight on a cholesterol-like molecule in the skin. Those living in high altitudes, who cover up their skin in sunlight or who stay indoors all day are not exposed to enough sunlight to meet their vitamin D needs. And once the UV index reduces to below 3, the skin reaction does not occur, so people living in northern climates are unable to synthesize their own vitamin D during most of the autumn and winter. Non-meat sources of vitamin D include mushrooms, eggs, fortified spreads, fortified cows' milk and soy milk, fortified cereals and butter.

Zinc

Zinc deficiency is common in people who don't eat meat. One of the earliest symptoms of zinc deficiency is loss of taste sensation. This forms the basis of a zinc-deficiency test that is widely available in pharmacies, and although it is not used by many orthodox nutritionists it is popular with nutritional therapists. A teaspoon of a solution of zinc sulphate (15 mg/5 ml concentration) is swirled in your mouth. If the solution seems tasteless, zinc deficiency is likely. If the solution tastes furry, of minerals or slightly sweet, zinc levels are borderline. If it tastes unpleasant, zinc levels are normal. Non-meat sources of zinc include brewer's yeast, wholegrains, nuts, seeds, dark green vegetables, pulses, eggs and cheese.

What a typical healthy vegetarian diet includes

The following list outlines an ideal vegetarian diet that will provide maximum micronutrients. Aim to eat:

- as wide a variety of foods as possible
- home-made rather than pre-packed or processed meals, which usually have reduced nutritional value (unless fortified)
- three to four servings of wholegrain products per day (e.g. bread, rice, pasta, buckwheat, polenta). These provide calories, protein, fibre, B vitamins, calcium and iron
- at least 400 g vegetables and/or fruit per day in total (five portions) for vitamins, minerals, antioxidants and other beneficial phytochemicals

- at least two pieces of fruit per day, one of which is a citrus fruit for vitamin C
- dried fruits for fibre and iron
- a large salad or portion of dark green leafy vegetables (e.g. spinach, watercress, broccoli, greens) per day for folate, calcium, iron and phytochemicals such as the carotenoid lutein
- nuts, seeds, pulses and cereals provide protein, although none contains all the essential amino acids together. These foods need to be mixed and matched – e.g. the essential amino acid missing from haricot beans is found in bread. Hence, combining cereals with pulses or seeds and nuts provides a balanced amino acid intake. Aim for two to three servings of pulses per day for protein, energy, fibre, calcium, iron, zinc and vitamin E and 30 g nuts and seeds per day
- two large portions of carrots or sweet potato (or yams) per week for antioxidant carotenoids such as betacarotene (which can be converted into vitamin A in the body)
- textured vegetable protein (TVP) made from soybeans as an excellent source of protein, calcium, iron, zinc, thiamin, riboflavin and niacin
- mycoprotein, derived from the fungus *Fusarium graminearum* as a good source of protein. Commercially available products can contain egg white, which is not suitable for vegans
- one pint of semi-skimmed milk (or fortified soy milk) per day for protein, calcium and trace minerals
- a serving of cheese per day for protein, calcium and minerals
- a total of three or four eggs per week for protein, D and B group vitamins, iron, selenium plus omega-3 fatty acids – especially from free-range birds fed an omega-enriched diet
- olive and rapeseed oils during cooking for important monounsaturated fats
- butter (scraped on bread) for vitamins D and E
- sources of vitamin B12, e.g. fortified soy milk, fortified breakfast cereals, fortified yeast extracts, Protoveg or supplements.

10

Nutrition and weight

For many people, over-nutrition is a big problem – and ironically this often goes hand in hand with a deficiency of key vitamins and minerals. Put simply, excess energy intake coupled with insufficient physical exercise leads to weight gain and, world-wide, obesity has more than doubled since 1980. According to the World Health Organization (WHO) that monitors global data, in 2008 1.5 billion adults aged 20 and over were overweight. Of these, 200 million men and nearly 300 million women were obese. This means that, overall, more than one in ten of the world's adult population is obese. In 2010, nearly 43 million children aged under five years were also overweight. These are harrowing figures, given the problems that obesity can lead to, and given that obesity is a totally preventable condition.

Our genetic time bomb

The genes that enabled cavemen to survive during conditions of alternating feast and famine are now working against us. Five hundred generations ago, when a large animal was killed, our primitive ancestors ate as much as they could in one go, as meat was less easy to preserve for future use as it is today. When gorging in this way, over a short period of time, the rapid conversion of dietary protein and fat into body-fat stores allowed for survival over the following days, weeks, or even months until the next significant source of food became available. Those whose genes promoted fat storage in this way survived better than those less genetically adapted to this way of life. Although food scarcity is still a problem in many parts of the world, affluent countries are battling with the opposite problem – an excess of calories, which our genes still store away for a future famine that never arrives. As a result, obesity rates are high – and increasing – in many countries, as shown in Table 20. In less affluent countries the rates are much lower. In India, for instance, only 9 per cent of adults are overweight and 2 per cent are obese.

Dietary excess is just as harmful to health as dietary lack, if not more so, as it increases the risk of life-shortening diseases such as coronary heart disease, stroke, Type 2 diabetes and some cancers. Conversely, as mentioned in the introduction to this book, a low-calorie intake is associated with longevity as long as there is no associated deficiency of vitamins and minerals.

Table 20 **Overweight and obesity rates in selected countries (collated 2010)**

Country	Prevalence of excess fat in adults	
	% overweight	% obese
Albania	49%	29%
Iceland	41%	18%
Germany	38%	21%
Australia	37%	25%
England	37%	25%
US	35%	34%
New Zealand	35%	25%
France	33%	17%
Bahrain	32%	27%

HEALTH RISKS OF OBESITY

Carrying excess weight is associated with high blood pressure, raised cholesterol levels, poor glucose tolerance and Type 2 diabetes, all of which, in turn, increase your risk of experiencing a heart attack or stroke.

- obesity doubles the risk of dying prematurely from coronary heart disease and stroke
- obesity increases the risk of Type 2 diabetes almost fortyfold, especially when excess fat is deposited around the abdomen and where weight is gained after the second decade of life – whatever the starting weight
- obesity doubles the risk of developing asthma
- someone who is obese will die, on average, seven years earlier than someone in the healthy weight range for their height
- severe obesity (BMI > 40 kg/M^2) is linked with up to a twelvefold increase in mortality among young adults compared to those who are in the healthy weight range for their height.

Your body-fat stores can be estimated using a calculation in which you divide your weight (in kilograms) by your height in metres and divide by your height again, as follows:

BMI = weight (kg) ÷ height (m) ÷ height (m)

This gives a number, called your Body Mass Index (BMI), which the World Health Organization interprets as follows:

WEIGHT BAND	BMI (kg/m^2)
Underweight	< 18.5
Normal range	18.5 to 24.9
Overweight (pre-obese)	25 to 29.9
Obese	> 30

You can find the ideal weight range for your height in Table 21, which is based on a BMI of 18.5 kg/M² to 24.9 kg/M² (calculations rounded up or down as appropriate).

Table 21 Ideal weight for height chart for adult men and women

Height		Optimum healthy weight range	
Metres	Feet	Kg	Stones
1.47	4' 10"	40.0–53.8	6 st 4 lb–8 st 6 lb
1.50	4' 11	41.6–56.0	6 st 8 lb–8 st 11 lb
1.52	5'	42.7–57.5	6 st 10–9 st
1.55	5' 1"	44.4–59.8	7 st–9 st 5 lb
1.57	5' 2"	45.6–61.4	7 st 2 lb–9 st 9 lb
1.60	5' 3"	47.4–63.7	7 st 6 lb–10 st
1.63	5' 4"	49.2–66.2	7 st 10 lb–10 st 5 lb
1.65	5' 5"	50.4–66.6	7 st 13 lb–10 st 7 lb
1.68	5' 6"	52.2–70.3	8 st 3 lb–11 st
1.70	5' 7"	53.5–72.0	8 st 6 lb–11 st 4 lb
1.73	5' 8"	55.4–74.5	8 st 10 lb–11 st 10 lb
1.75	5' 9"	56.7–76.3	8 st 13 lb–12 st
1.78	5' 10"	58.6–78.9	9 st 3 lb–12 st 5 lb
1.80	5' 11"	60.0–80.7	9 st 6 lb–12 st 9 lb
1.83	6'	62.0–83.4	9 st 10 lb–13 st 1 lb
1.85	6' 1"	63.3–85.2	9 st 13 lb–13 st 5 lb
1.88	6' 2"	65.4–88.0	10 st 4 lb–13 st 11 lb
1.90	6' 3"	66.8–89.9	10 st 7 lb–14 st 1 lb
1.93	6' 4"	68.9–92.8	10 st 12 lb–14 st 8 lb

But it's not just the quantity of excess fat you 'own' – where you store it is also important. People who inherit genes that deposit excess fat around the internal organs (known as visceral, central, truncal, apple-shaped or android obesity) are more likely to develop health problems than those who store fat around their hips (pear-shaped). This is because visceral fat is different from fat stored elsewhere in the body. It secretes hormones and free fatty acids that travel directly to your liver, where they activate genes that increase liver production of cholesterol, clotting factors and other inflammatory mediators. They also act as a signal that fat stores are full, so cells become resistant to the effects of insulin and less glucose can enter cells. In addition, when free fatty-acid levels are high, muscle cells use them as a fuel, so they burn less glucose, while liver cells use them to produce new glucose – all of these factors can contribute to impaired glucose tolerance.

For Asian men, the health risks are greatest when their waist circumference expands to greater than 90 cm (36"), while for Asian women risks increase significantly above a waist size of 80 cm (32"). For people of other ethnic origins, the risk is highest once waist size reaches 102 cm (40") for men or 88 cm (35") for women. Different figures arise because research has shown that Asian men and women tend to have a higher proportion of body fat to muscle than the rest of the UK population and also tend to store fat around their middle. These genetic differences lead to a greater risk of developing Type 2 diabetes and coronary heart disease at a lower waist size than people of other ethnic backgrounds.

To some extent, obesity is hereditary. If both your parents are obese, you have a 70 per cent chance of obesity too, compared with less than 20 per cent if both parents are lean. This isn't just a question of inheriting bad genes, though; family eating habits and activity patterns are also predictors of weight gain.

Appetite versus hunger

Although doctors used to dismiss the idea that hormone imbalances could cause obesity, new research suggests that this is in fact the case. It's not the traditional hormones that are involved, however, but newly identified substances produced by your intestinal and fat cells that influence the satiety centre in your brain. Unravelling how these hormones work, and their potential as treatments for obesity and diabetes, is one of the most important areas of nutritional research today, as the development of new drugs could help to treat or prevent the current epidemic in obesity.

Ghrelin is a hormone produced by cells in the lining of an empty stomach. Ghrelin directly stimulates your appetite centre in the hypothalamus of the brain to produce feelings of hunger. Infusing ghrelin into the circulation has been shown to increase food intake by as much as 28 per cent. Once you start to eat, however, ghrelin levels soon fall. Eating a high glycaemic-load breakfast (e.g. white toast, sugary cereal, sweetened orange juice) lowers ghrelin levels by 41 per cent; eating a low glycaemic-load breakfast (e.g. wholegrain muesli, boiled egg, unsweetened grapefruit juice) reduces ghrelin levels by 33 per cent, while a low-calorie breakfast lowers ghrelin by just 24 per cent. The fall in ghrelin levels is linked with increasing levels of insulin, and it was recently recognized that ghrelin may help to control glucose metabolism.

Obestatin hormone is so closely related to ghrelin that it's coded for by the same stretch of DNA, and its existence was deduced using computer analysis of the ghrelin gene. Researchers believe that the gene codes for a protein splits to produce both ghrelin and obestatin. Obestatin is believed to counteract ghrelin and reduce hunger. Latest research suggests that impaired control of the ghrelin-obestatin system may trigger obesity and diabetes.

Leptin hormone is produced by overstuffed adipose (fat) cells in an attempt to reduce food intake. The amount of leptin you produce is directly related to the size of your fat stores, so you'd expect that the more you weigh, the fuller you'd feel. Unfortunately, there's a catch: as you get more and more overweight, leptin receptors in the appetite centre of your brain become less and less responsive to its effects. The satiety signal that stops you eating simply doesn't get through. This effect is linked with insulin resistance, and people with Type 2 diabetes have higher leptin levels than those without, whether or not they are also overweight. In fact, leptin appears to be involved in insulin secretion, and having a high leptin level may predict who will go on to develop diabetes, as the development of leptin resistance appears to precede the development of insulin resistance. Regular exercise may reduce leptin resistance as well as improve insulin resistance through its effects on muscle and fat metabolism.

Cholecystokinin (CCK) is a hormone produced in your small intestine (duodenum) when partially digested protein and fats are squirted through from the stomach. CCK acts on your gall bladder to stimulate release of bile. It also acts as a signal of satiety for the brain so you stop eating. CCK boosts the effects of leptin, and these two hormones may interact synergistically to control long-term food intake. If you chew your food thoroughly, and pause between mouthfuls, this will slow down your eating and give your brain more time to receive the CCK signal that you are full.

Glucagon-like peptide-1 (GLP-1) is a hormone released towards the end of your small intestine (ileum) as yet another signal to reduce hunger and food intake. Interestingly, GLP-1 also stimulates release of insulin, and this effect is preserved in people with Type 2 diabetes. However, the release of GLP-1 after a carbohydrate-rich meal is lower in people who are obese than in those who are lean, which may be a genetic effect.

Oxyntomodulin is another hormone produced in the lower small intestine (ileum) and also in the colon. Circulating levels of oxyntomodulin rise within 30 minutes of eating and remain elevated for several hours. It's thought to work on the appetite centre of the brain, and oxyntomodulin infusion can reduce food intake by 20 per cent and levels of ghrelin by over 40 per cent.

Peptide-YY (PYY) and Pancreatic Polypeptide (PP) are also satiety hormones released from the ileum and colon shortly after food intake. A virtually identical hormone, pancreatic polypeptide (PP) is released from the pancreas after eating, and suppresses appetite throughout most of the day. People who are obese have lower than normal levels of both hormones. Infusions of PYY can reduce food intake by 33 per cent over a 24-hour period, while those given an infusion of PP consumed 22 per cent fewer calories at an eat-all-you-can buffet two hours later.

Cortisol is a stress hormone released from the adrenal glands during times of physical and emotional stress. It may be linked with a stress response in which you increase food intake (comfort eating). In one study, women were exposed to stressful activities and then left alone to recover with a bowl of snacks (but didn't know their food intake was being investigated). Those whose cortisol level increased significantly in response to stress ate an average of 216 kcal afterwards, while those who coped better, and showed a lower cortisol reaction, snacked less (137 kcal). Those who responded to stress with high cortisol levels also showed a preference for sweet rather than salty snacks. On the control day, when they were not stressed, however, both groups ate similar amounts of snacks (177 kcal versus 187 kcal). This suggests that some people respond to stress by eating more, while others eat less, and cortisol may be involved. Eating and appetite is a complex behaviour: long-term stress may influence eating behaviour and lead to noticeable weight gain in some people. Exercise helps to overcome the effects of cortisol by resetting the flight-or-fight stress reaction to the rest-and-digest response. Exercise also boosts fat burning, reduces insulin resistance and triggers release of endorphins – brain chemicals that suppress hunger and increase feelings of euphoria.

The interaction between different hormones has a profound effect on hunger and food intake. What's more, appetite control is closely linked with obesity, insulin resistance and diabetes. Despite the abundance of appetite-suppressing hormones in the body (obestatin, leptin, cholecystokinin, glucagon-like peptide-1, oxyntomodulin, peptide-YY, pancreatic polypeptide), the only two that markedly stimulate appetite – ghrelin and cortisol – seem to win every time.

Losing weight

Your daily energy requirement depends on your age, sex, level of activity and occupation, and is discussed in Chapter 3, where you will also find Table 8, which shows the average daily energy needs for men and women. Put simply, to lose excess weight, you will need to consume less energy than you need so that the deficit is met by raiding the fat deposited in your adipose stores.

Losing weight reduces your risk of developing Type 2 diabetes by as much as 58 per cent, as it improves insulin resistance and glucose tolerance. Losing just 10 kg (22 lb) in weight can reduce fasting blood-glucose levels by 50 per cent, as well as lowering blood pressure by an average of 10/20 mmHg, triglycerides by 30 per cent and harmful LDL cholesterol by 15 per cent, while increasing 'good' HDL-cholesterol by at least 8 per cent. As a result, for someone who is obese, losing 10 kg can reduce their overall risk of premature death by 20 per cent and the risk of a diabetes-related death by as much as 30 per cent. Even slight waist reductions of just 5 cm to 10 cm can considerably reduce your risk of a heart attack.

Types of diet

The vast majority of weight-loss diets fall into five main types: low-calorie diets, very low-calorie diets, low-fat diets, low-carbohydrate/high protein diets and low glycaemic-index diets.

Low-calorie

Low-calorie diets providing 1,000 to 1,500 kcal per day are effective for weight loss if they are followed long term, for at least six months, and can achieve an average weight loss of 8 per cent over a six- to twelve-month period. For someone weighing 100 kg, that represents a weight loss of 8 kg. It is easy to underestimate your calorie intake, however, and this method should ideally involve weighing foods, at least initially, to help you understand portion control (for example, the size of a piece of cheese that provides 120 kcal energy is smaller than most people realize). Studies that have looked at long-term outcomes and the ability to keep weight off suggest that they are less effective, though, as after three to four years the average weight loss is half that seen in shorter-term trials, at around 4 per cent of body weight (equivalent to just 4 kg for someone with a starting weight of 100 kg). These diets depend on constant vigilance and record-keeping, which is difficult to maintain long term.

Very low-calorie

Very low-calorie diets typically provide between 400 and 800 kcal per day, in the form of fortified, sweet or savoury drinks that replace between one and three meals per day. These provide the vitamins and minerals you need but restrict your energy intake. Under professional supervision, these diets can help you lose between 13 kg to 23 kg excess weight over the course of 12 to 18 weeks. Although these diets used to be considered extreme, they are now gaining medical acceptance for some people as part of an ongoing, structured, educational and behavioural support programme to change long-term eating and lifestyle habits. A meta-analysis of 29 studies investigating how well people managed to keep excess weight off, once they had lost it, found that very low-calorie diets were much more successful than a traditional calorie-controlled or low-fat diet, and helped people keep off considerably more weight at every year of follow-up – even up to five years.

NB These diets are considered safe and effective but only when used by appropriately selected individuals (usually with a BMI of 30 kg/M^2 or greater) under careful medical supervision. Do not follow this approach on your own. However, a modified form of VLCD is currently popular, known as the 5:2, or intermittent fasting diet, in which you eat a normal healthy diet for five days, and restrict calories to 500 (women) to 600 (men) calories for two days. This can safely be followed on your own.

Low-fat

Low-fat diets were originally based on the idea that, as fat supplies twice as many calories per gram as either protein or carbohydrate, cutting back on fat will cut back on calorie intake more effectively than cutting back on other food groups. Low-fat diets involve restricting your total fat intake to less than 30 per cent of energy intake, with reduction in saturated fat – typically to less than 7 per cent daily energy. In comparison, a typical Western diet provides over 35 per cent of energy in the form of fat, with 10 per cent or more calories coming from saturated fat. Moderate consumption of monounsaturated fats (olive and rapeseed oils) is encouraged, as are wholegrain carbohydrates, but refined and simple sugars are avoided. Although low-fat diets are the traditional weight-loss tools recommended by healthcare professionals, large studies suggest that low-fat diets are no better than low-calorie diets in helping people to achieve long-term weight loss, and that it is the energy restriction that helps weight loss rather than the fact that the diet is low in fat per se. After six months, average weight loss is around 5 kg in those following a low-fat diet, and 6.5 kg in those on a low-calorie diet. After 18 months, those following a low-fat diet have usually gained 0.1 kg from their starting weight, while those following a low-calorie diet tend to maintain a weight loss of 2.3 kg.

Low-fat diets are also promoted to help lower cholesterol levels and reduce the risk of coronary heart disease. However, the quality of fat consumed is just as important as the quantity, and a recent meta-analysis of six trials has shown that a high-fat Mediterranean diet improves heart-disease risk factors such as blood pressure, glucose control and cholesterol balance more effectively than a low-fat diet.

Low-carbohydrate/high-protein

Low-carbohydrate/high-protein diets can produce notable weight loss over six months, typically in the region of 7 per cent of body weight. This is partly because protein fills you up quickly and involves the expenditure of significant amounts of energy during its metabolism, and partly because a low-carbohydrate diet reduces secretion of insulin – your body's main fat-storing hormone. 'Celebrity' regimes based on this approach such as the Atkins, South Beach and Dukan diets have gained huge popularity. A huge meta-analysis of 87 studies published in the *American Journal of Clinical Nutrition* in 2006 found that, after diets providing less than the usually recommended 45 to 65 per cent of carbohydrate were associated with a 2.05 kg greater loss of fat mass than diets supplying a higher percentage of energy from carbohydrate over a period of at least four weeks. Although high-protein/low-carbohydrate diets are effective for weight loss over the short term, their long-term benefits are still uncertain and they remain controversial. In addition, many people do not follow them correctly, and do not eat the large amount of salad and green leafy vegetables recommended, which can lead to problems such as constipation.

Low glycaemic

The Comprehensive Assessment of Long-term Effects of Reducing Intake of Energy (CALERIE) trial carried out at the Tufts-New England Medical Center and published in *Diabetes Care*, the journal of the American Diabetes Association, found that overweight people with a higher insulin secretion lost more weight on a low glycaemic-load diet (40 per cent carbohydrate, 30 per cent fat, average daily glycaemic index 53) compared with a high glycaemic-load diet (60 per cent carbohydrate, 20 per cent fat, average daily glycaemic index 86). The target energy intake in both groups was 1,966 kcal per day. Those with high insulin levels lost around 10 kg weight on the low glycaemic diet compared with around 6 kg on the high glycaemic diet. A low GI diet improves satiety and appears to promote weight loss, compared with a high-carbohydrate diet – probably because it reduces secretion of insulin, which is the main fat-storing hormone in the body. There is a growing consensus that a low glycaemic diet that emphazises monounsaturated fats is the diet of choice for people with insulin resistance, metabolic syndrome or diabetes.

Meal replacement

These provide nutritionally balanced shakes, soups, protein-rich bars, low glycaemic index bars or portion-controlled ready meals for reheating in a pouch. These products are intended to replace one, two or occasionally three meals per day, as well as providing nutritious snacks. They ensure you obtain all the vitamins and minerals you need in a format that may be calorie-, fat- and/or sugar-controlled. Meal-replacement products can be successful for people who live busy lives and would otherwise grab an unhealthy fat or sugar-laden snack when away from home. They are also useful for people who tend to eat alone, or who would otherwise have to prepare a separate 'diet' meal for themselves while also feeding a growing family.

Whatever eating pattern you choose to follow, it is important to stick with it until you have reached a healthy weight for your height. Once your goal is attained, you then need to ensure you don't slowly regain the lost weight. For most people, the types of diet that are easiest to follow long-term are usually a balanced, calorie-controlled diet and a diet that provides complex carbohydrates and lots of fruit and vegetables, such as the Mediterranean diet or a low glycaemic-load diet.

Small eating changes to help you lose weight

The following general weight-loss tips will help:

- *Always eat breakfast* to kick-start your metabolism so that you burn up more energy. A growing number of studies show that consuming breakfast helps to reduce weight gain in children, adolescents and adults.
- *Drink a glass of water before eating* to stop you mistaking thirst for hunger, and to help you fill up.
- *Always sit down at a laid table to eat*, don't eat 'on the hoof' while standing up and walking around or you will not appreciate what you are eating and may eat more.

Use a smaller plate to trick your brain into thinking you are eating more than you are.

Don't leave serving dishes on the table or you are likely to help yourself to too much – and go back for seconds.

Serve smaller helpings than you think you need.

Fill your plate with naturally colourful foods that are high in vitamins, minerals and fibre, such as red, green and yellow vegetables and salad stuff. A good rule is that the more colours, the more the variety of nutrients.

Chew each mouthful for longer to give your brain more time to receive signals that you are becoming full.

Pause regularly while eating so your meal lasts longer, and you start to feel full up before you've eaten too much.

Concentrate on enjoying your food – focus on the flavour rather than reading or TV, or you may end up eating more without realizing it.

Purposely leave some food on your plate: don't scrape your plate clean.

Wait to eat – to train yourself to tell hunger and appetite apart, force yourself to wait an extra 15 to 20 minutes whenever you fancy a snack. If it is appetite, the urge will disappear. If it is true hunger, sit down at the table and eat a healthy snack.

Keep a food diary and write down everything you eat – this is especially helpful when you find it difficult to lose weight.

Nutrition is an evolving science, and what we think we know now, and our current best-advice guidelines, may change as the study of nutrigenomics – the interactions between our food and our genes – evolves.

In the meantime, most people would benefit from looking more closely at the quality, quantity and balance of what they eat and drink. Even if you only make one or two small changes to improve the nutrient profile of your diet, you are likely to gain long-term benefits. Like all ingrained habits, maintaining dietary changes is never easy. To accomplish changes long-term, it's usually best to tackle things slowly. The Japanese have a useful philosophy known as *kaizen*, which essentially means committing yourself to make continuous small steps towards improvement. This is the ideal way to address your diet. Small changes might include eating an extra portion of vegetables per week, or cutting out meat on one day, or even eating less every other day.

Enjoy your food.

Resources and further reading

Useful websites

American Dietetic Association www.eatright.org
United States Department of Agriculture's Food and Nutrition Information
    Center www.nutrition.gov
Dieticians of Canada www.dietitians.ca
British Nutrition Foundation www.nutrition.org.uk
The Nutrition Society www.nutritionsociety.org
British Dietetic Association www.bda.uk.com

Introductory books

Denby, N., Baic, S., Rinzler, C.A. *Nutrition for Dummies*. Hoboken, New
    Jersey, John Wiley & Sons, second edition, 2010
Geissler, C., Powers, H. *Fundamentals of Human Nutrition: for Students and
    Practitioners in the Health Sciences*. Philadelphia, Churchill Livingstone,
    2009
Gibney, M. J., Lanham-New, S.A., Cassidy, A., Vorster, H. H. *Introduction
    to Human Nutrition (The Nutrition Society Textbook)*. Hoboken, New
    Jersey, Wiley-Blackwell, second edition, 2009

Comprehensive textbooks

Erdman, J.W. Jr, MacDonald, I.A., Zeisel, S.H. (eds) *Present Knowledge in
    Nutrition*. New Jersey, Wiley-Blackwell, tenth edition, 2012

Lanham-New, S.A., Macdonald, I.A., Roche, H.M. *Nutrition and Metabolism (The Nutrition Society Textbook)*. Hoboken, New Jersey, Wiley-Blackwell, second edition, 2010

Salway, J. G., *Metabolism at a Glance*. Hoboken, New Jersey, Wiley-Blackwell, third edition, 2003

Stargrove, M.B., Treasure, J., McKee, D.L. *Herb, Nutrient and Drug Interactions: Clinical Implications and Therapeutic Strategies*. Philadelphia, Mosby, 2008

Textbook of Functional Medicine. Washington, Institute for Functional Medicine, 2006

Index

Note: *t* following a page number denotes a table.